Baby-led Breastfeeding

How to make breastfeeding work with your baby's help

GILL RAPLEY & TRACEY MURKETT

Vermilion
LONDON

1 3 5 7 9 10 8 6 4 2

Published in 2012 by Vermilion, an imprint of Ebury Publishing
Ebury Publishing is a Random House Group company

The Random House Group Limited Reg. No. 954009
Addresses for companies within the Random House Group can be found at
www.randomhouse.co.uk

A CIP catalogue record for this book is available from the British Library

The Random House Group Limited supports The Forest Stewardship Council (FSC®),
the leading international forest certification organisation. Our books carrying the FSC
label are printed on FSC® certified paper. FSC is the only forest certification scheme
endorsed by the leading environmental organisations, including Greenpeace. Our
paper procurement policy can be found at www.randomhouse.co.uk/environment

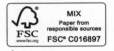

MIX
Paper from
responsible sources
FSC® C016897

Printed and bound by CPI Group (UK) Ltd, Croydon, CR0 4YY

ISBN 9780091935290

Copies are available at special rates for bulk orders. Contact the sales development
team on 020 7840 8487 for more information.

To buy books by your favourite authors and register for offers, visit
www.randomhouse.co.uk

This book is dedicated to the memory of
Tracey's mother, Ivy, and her sister, Sally,
who both championed breastfeeding long
before Tracey had the chance to discover why.

Contents

Introduction

Breastfeeding is important. It protects against illness, promotes optimal development and helps to build a strong and lasting bond between mother and baby – laying the foundation for a lifetime's good health and emotional wellbeing. It's the natural and normal way to feed a baby.

Yet you are likely to come across an enormous amount of conflicting advice and information about breastfeeding from friends and relatives, in websites and books – and even from health professionals. Much of this advice (and the out-dated practices still common in some hospitals) actually makes breastfeeding *more difficult*. Separating a mother from her baby, imposing parent-led routines, and taking a rigid approach to feeding positions can all interfere with the way a woman's body produces milk.

As a result, many mothers find that breastfeeding is painful or stressful, instead of the joy it should be. More than a third of UK mothers who start breastfeeding have changed to formula by the time their baby is just six weeks old; most had stopped before they planned to and many are bitterly disappointed. But the root of most of the common problems is the same – they're caused by struggling against the baby's instincts.

Baby-led breastfeeding is based on how breastfeeding *really* **works.** It centres on trusting babies to know what they need. It recognises their innate skills and the powerful effects of hormones and instincts in both mother and baby. And it works *with* those skills and instincts, rather than fighting against them.

This book explains why following your baby's lead makes sense and shows you how to let him use his instincts to help you to breastfeed. It will give you the information and practical tips you need to enjoy relaxed and stress-free feeding for as long as you both want – whether this is your first baby, you've struggled with breastfeeding in the past or you've only ever used formula.

Baby-led Breastfeeding is the book we wish we'd had when our babies were little. Between us we made all sorts of mistakes and encountered a variety of problems. Our experiences since then, as a health professional (Gill) and as voluntary breastfeeding supporters (both of us), have convinced us that babies really do know what they're doing, and that responding to them is the key to getting breastfeeding to work. We hope this book will give you the confidence to trust your baby and follow his lead, so that breastfeeding is happy and rewarding for you both.

Note

Throughout the book when referring to the baby we have alternated between 'he' and 'she', chapter by chapter, to be fair to both sexes. And although the information is relevant for both fathers and mothers, we've addressed the reader as the mother, for ease of understanding.

---

part I

The basics of baby-led breastfeeding

1

Thinking about breastfeeding

Baby-led breastfeeding is all about allowing your baby to use his instincts and understanding how you can help your body to respond to his needs, so that you can both enjoy relaxed and stress-free breastfeeding.

There isn't really much you need to do in terms of preparation and, in a sense, you don't even have to make a decision to breastfeed beforehand, because if you are led by your baby he will instinctively want to feed from your breast. However, it can help to know why breastfeeding is considered so important. This chapter aims to provide you with some of those facts, plus some tips on what to expect and what you can do in advance to help things go smoothly.

Is breast really best?

Breastfeeding is the biologically normal way to feed human babies. All babies are born with the instinct to do it and all mothers have milk in their breasts by the time their baby arrives. So it seems a bit odd to talk about the *benefits* of breastfeeding. We don't talk about the benefits of breathing clean air or drinking clean water – we talk about the *risks* of breathing polluted air or drinking dirty water. So it's more accurate to talk about the risks of *not* breastfeeding. Because

5

of advances in formula manufacture, these risks aren't as big as they were; but they're there, even so. And a growing amount of research means that we now know more about them, and they're getting harder to ignore.

Most people know that breastmilk contains everything a baby needs and that it's always at the right temperature. But there's a lot more to it than that. Research shows that whether babies have breastmilk or formula really does make a difference – not just while they're babies, or children, but throughout their lives, whether their parents are rich or poor, wherever they live in the world and whatever their family medical history (see UNICEF, *Sources of information and support*, page 279).

Illnesses that are more common in babies and children who were formula fed

- Gastroenteritis (vomiting and diarrhoea)
- Necrotising enterocolitis (a very serious infection of the gut, which occurs mainly in premature babies)
- Chest infections and wheezing conditions
- Eczema
- Middle ear infections and 'glue ear'
- Urinary tract infections
- Sudden Infant Death Syndrome (also known as 'cot death')
- Leukaemia.

And when they grow up ...

- Obesity
- High blood pressure
- High cholesterol levels
- Diabetes.

It's not just a question of coughs and colds but serious conditions, such as diabetes and leukaemia. The box on page 6 lists illnesses for which there is good evidence of a link with formula feeding as a baby.

The secret lies not so much in the nutrients in breastmilk (which can be mimicked reasonably well in formula), but in its other ingredients (which can't). Breastmilk protects babies partly through antibodies, which protect against infections, and partly through factors that support the baby's immature organs, helping them to mature quickly and function well, and making them more resistant to disease. The action of feeding at the breast is also important: a breastfed baby's mouth develops differently from the mouth of a baby who is bottle fed. Not only are breastfed babies less likely than formula-fed babies to get infectious illnesses, they're also *more* likely to have straight teeth.

Amazing antibodies

Breastmilk contains antibodies that protect the baby from infections the mother has had (or been immunised against) in the past, such as rubella (German measles). But her body is also continually making new antibodies as it detects germs in the air around her and in her food – and it sends them straight to the breast, to be added to her milk. So her baby is protected at his very next feed. This continual updating (like a computer's virus checker) means that breastfed babies are much less likely to catch common infections such as colds, flu and tummy bugs – as well as more serious illnesses – than babies who are not breastfed.

Breastfeeding isn't just good for babies – it's good for mothers, too

Women who breastfeed have less chance of developing breast and ovarian cancers than those who don't. Breastfeeding seems to help reset the mother's metabolism, too, allowing it to return more easily to the way it was before pregnancy, resulting in higher calcium levels (reducing the chance of osteoporosis and hip fractures in old age) and effective insulin production (which makes the development of diabetes less likely). Breastfeeding also helps the womb to return to its non-pregnant size (see page 25) and has a contraceptive effect (see page 136).

Of course, breastfeeding doesn't *guarantee* good health but it does make it more likely. And *not* breastfeeding doesn't always lead to illness – but it does increase the risk. The more breastmilk your baby has, and the longer you breastfeed for, the greater the health protection you both gain. Giving nothing but breastmilk for the first six months, and continuing to breastfeed well beyond your child's first birthday, is the way to maximise the advantages for both of you.

'I love the feeling that this child is growing big and strong and beautiful because of what I'm doing – it's all my milk. I know I'm giving him the best start that I can.'

Becky, mother of Jack, five months

It's not just about the milk

In the same way that *breastmilk* is about more than nutrition, *breastfeeding* is about more than satisfying hunger. The breastfeeding relationship is special, personal and unique – different for every mother and baby. It gives babies much more than food.

Breastfeeding involves close contact. This closeness means that you and your baby are communicating throughout every breastfeed, even if you don't say a word. Your nipple and your baby's mouth are both very sensitive, with lots of nerve endings, and your baby is near enough while he's feeding to hear your heart beating. Together, you pick up even the slightest movements and mood changes in each other. Of course, you can hold your baby very close while bottle feeding – but it's not an intrinsic part of feeding in the way it is with breastfeeding.

Breastfeeding mothers and their babies are attuned to each other on a deep biological level. In fact, a breastfeeding mother and her baby are sometimes referred to as a 'dyad' – two individuals so closely linked they are considered one unit. Her body nourishes him; his feeding determines her milk production (see page 25). He relies on her for food; she relies on him to keep her breasts producing milk without becoming uncomfortably full.

Most people know it's important for mothers and babies to bond and that breastfeeding can play an important role in this. A strong bond between mother and baby makes the baby feel secure and loved, and ensures that his mother cares for him. Bonding isn't unique to breastfeeding – formula-fed babies bond with their mothers too. But, because of the hormones it triggers (see *The role of the 'love' hormone*, page 24), breastfeeding provides a shortcut to bonding.

Bonding is not only good for babies' development and happiness; it also makes parenting easier. The hormones of breastfeeding make a mother want to respond to her baby and help her to interpret his needs. And, because it provides pretty much everything a healthy newborn could want (apart from a clean nappy!), breastfeeding makes parenting less stressful and tiring than it would otherwise be.

A breastfeeding mother who is following her baby's lead can often sense when he is going to want to feed – and she doesn't need to decide whether he's hungry, thirsty or just a bit miserable, nor how much milk to give. She can also offer him a quick snack now and then, to help her fit his feeds around her other commitments. This level of flexibility isn't available with formula feeding.

Research also shows that breastfeeding mothers get more restful sleep than those who bottle feed, especially if they keep their babies near them at night. This isn't just because the baby doesn't have to wait for the feed to be prepared; it's because the hormones of breastfeeding are designed to make both of them feel relaxed and woozy, helping them to go back to sleep quickly.

Finally, let's not forget that – when it's going smoothly – breastfeeding *feels* nice! Most mothers find it soothing. Some say it gives them a warm 'glow'. Others say it makes them feel relaxed and slightly 'spaced out'. This feel-good factor is a natural part of breastfeeding and the special closeness that it brings.

'I find breastfeeding really enjoyable – I love the feeling of Evie being on my breast, the close physical contact, and her lying in my arms. She's almost three now – hopefully she'll have memories of being close to her mum when she was little.'

Maria, *mother of Evie, two years*

Why doesn't everyone breastfeed?

Although most people now know that 'breast is best', in many western countries – including the UK – formula feeding has become the usual way to feed babies. A key reason for this is that, until relatively recently, the advice mothers were given about how to breastfeed actually made it more difficult for them. Practices such as feeding 'by the clock' (every four hours for ten minutes on each breast) and separating babies from their mothers at night were commonplace until the 1980s. Restricting breastfeeding and mother–baby contact like this is almost guaranteed to prevent mothers from making enough milk for their babies, so many women found that, within a few weeks, they had to resort to formula. As a result, several generations of women believed they 'couldn't breastfeed' and, over time, formula feeding became the norm.

Another piece of the jigsaw is the fact that many parents today don't live close to their extended family so, even in families where breastfeeding is usual, many children grow up without ever having seen it done. All of this means that knowledge about breastfeeding is no longer passed down through the generations in the way it once was and formula feeding is often taken for granted.

Will I be able to breastfeed?

Many women worry whether they have the right type of breast (or nipple) for breastfeeding. **The size and shape of your breasts will only affect how you hold your baby for feeding – they won't make any difference to how much milk you produce.** It doesn't matter, either, whether your nipples are large, small, prominent, flat or inverted (tucked inwards instead of pointing outwards), because babies don't feed by sucking on the nipple; they take a big mouthful of breast (see *Getting the angle right*, page 36). Gadgets on the market designed to help nipples stand out are for cosmetic purposes only – they aren't necessary for breastfeeding.

Although all kinds of nipples and breasts will 'work' for breastfeeding, the following circumstances can sometimes give rise to concerns:

- *Pierced nipples* don't usually cause a problem with breastfeeding. Occasionally, nipple piercings cause some of the milk ducts to seal over, so milk can't get out from those sections of the breast. If this happens, milk production will stop in those areas and the rest of the breast will produce more. You should remove any rings or bars before you feed, though, so they don't hurt your baby's mouth, or you may prefer to let the holes close and have your nipples re-pierced later.

- *Implants* (to increase the size of the breasts) are inserted behind the milk-making tissue, so they don't interfere with milk production or with the baby getting milk out. Some women who have had implants find that their breasts are a bit tight, making them uncomfortable very quickly if feeding is delayed. You can prevent this by encouraging your baby to feed frequently and by hand expressing your milk whenever he has a longer gap.

- *Breast surgery* can affect breastfeeding, depending on the reason for the operation and the way it was carried out. Surgery to remove a breast lump usually causes damage to the ducts, but only in one area of the breast. The rest of the breast (and the other breast) will work quite normally. After a mastectomy it's usually possible to fully breastfeed from the remaining breast. However, you should check with your surgeon whether the reason for the surgery, or any other treatment it involved, might mean that breastfeeding is not advisable.

- *Breast reduction* usually relies on removal of fat tissue (rather than milk-making tissue) but sometimes it involves cutting the milk ducts and the nerves that supply the nipple. If your nipples have been re-sited – and especially if they are no longer sensitive – breastfeeding may be difficult. Surgery to alter the shape of the nipples can have the same effect. However, breastfeeding *can* work after surgery and even if you can't breastfeed your baby fully, he may be able to have some of your milk.

How do I prepare?

There are a few things you can do while you're pregnant to get ready for breastfeeding. For example, taking some time to learn how breastfeeding works and how you can help your baby follow his instincts, and to think about how a new baby will fit into your family, will make things easier for all of you.

It's good to be ready for any stories of breastfeeding failure you come across, from friends, family or in the media, which can be demoralising. Almost all women *can* breastfeed – but the wrong advice, especially early on, is sometimes all it takes to make it very difficult. An understanding of what your baby needs to do, and respect for his and your instincts, will help you decide which suggestions are going to be helpful and which may lead to problems.

'All the way through my pregnancy Paul went on about "When life gets back to normal ..." I don't think either of us realised life would never be the same again. I had more of an idea than him, though – he really wasn't ready for it!'

Anna, mother of Joseph, 20 months

Anticipating a change in lifestyle

Some people imagine that breastfeeding is very time-consuming. This is true in the early weeks, while you are both learning, when it can take more time than bottle feeding. However, as mother and baby get more skilled it becomes quicker and easier, and from about six weeks onwards (sometimes earlier), breastfeeding is much less hassle than using formula.

Whichever way you feed your baby, the first few weeks are a period of huge adjustment. Many expectant women find it hard to imagine just how much their baby will need them and how urgent his needs will be, day and night. When a baby needs his mother it's impossible for him to wait patiently, even for a few minutes, because he only understands the way he feels *now*. Some of the things you currently take for granted (such as being able to spend an hour cooking a meal) may benefit from a bit of re-thinking, so that you'll be able to interrupt what you're doing easily to feed him.

Breastfeeding will work best if you keep your baby close to you, especially in the first few hours and days, and let him lead the way. It's important that your main supporter (whether that's your partner, your mother or a close friend) understands how much this matters and the difference it will make to how easy or difficult you find breastfeeding. He or she will have a crucial role to play in protecting you and your baby from other people who may – with the best will in the world – want to suggest things that could interfere with your chances of problem-free feeding.

Preparing your breasts – what you need to do (or not)

In the past, women were told they should do certain things to their breasts towards the end of pregnancy to get them ready for breastfeeding. They were advised to toughen up their nipples, to do 'exercises' (or wear devices called breast shells) if their nipples were inverted, and to express a little milk now and then to clear out the ducts. All of this is unnecessary. In fact, a mother's breasts prepare perfectly well for breastfeeding all by themselves (see box, opposite).

Rubbing your nipples or applying strong ointments may be harmful, causing pain and damaging sensitive skin. You don't need tough nipples to breastfeed and there are no treatments or creams that will prevent you from getting sore – only attention to how your baby feeds can do that (see Chapter 3).

It *is* a good idea, though, to avoid using soap on your breasts, and anything that could make your skin extra-sensitive or mask your natural smell (for example, perfumed bath products), towards the end of your pregnancy.

How your body prepares for breastfeeding

As soon as you become pregnant, your body starts to get ready for breastfeeding. For many women, tender breasts – caused by the changes happening inside them – are the first sign that a baby is on the way. Here's what's going on:

- The network of blood vessels that supplies your breasts is expanding, helping them to prepare for milk making. Some of these blood vessels may show through your skin, giving an effect known as 'marbling'.
- The milk-producing cells in your breast (see page 22) are multiplying rapidly. If you've had a baby before, a few of the cells you made in that pregnancy will still be there – but mostly it's a whole new batch.
- You'll notice your nipples and areolas (the dark skin around your nipples) gradually getting darker and more sensitive – and your nipples may stand out more.
- You may notice small bumps on the skin around your nipples. These are glands known as Montgomery's tubercles. They produce an oil that keeps the skin clean and supple and has a smell unique to you, which will help your baby to recognise you and trigger his instincts for feeding.
- From about 16 weeks of pregnancy your breasts will start to produce colostrum, a thick, sticky fluid that looks a bit like honey. This is concentrated breastmilk (see *The first milk*, page 27). It may leak, or form a dry layer on the tips of your nipples, or you may be able to squeeze a bit out (see below). Or you may not be aware of it at all.

Expressing colostrum during pregnancy can be a useful way to learn how to hand express (see page 86) – or to reassure yourself that your breasts are doing what they're supposed to (and that your nipples really do have holes in the ends!) – but it isn't necessary and it won't affect your ability to breastfeed. The exception to this is if you know your baby is going to be born early, or if you have a condition such as diabetes (see page 67). In that case your midwife may suggest that you express and freeze your colostrum from about 36 weeks of pregnancy onwards, in case your baby needs extra when he's born. Every time you express colostrum, more is made, so there's no need to worry that you'll use it up.

What to buy – or not

Although it can be tempting to buy lots of equipment ready for your new baby, there's really very little you need for breastfeeding – nature has equipped you with the most important items. There are some extras, though, that may make life easier.

Do I need a breastfeeding bra?

You don't have to buy special nursing bras for breastfeeding and, if you don't normally wear a bra, there's no reason to feel you have to buy one just because you're planning to breastfeed. However, your breasts will be heavier than usual at times (including while you're pregnant), so you may welcome some extra support. A bra is also useful for holding breast pads (see page 18).

It's best to get yourself properly fitted, especially if you have large breasts. Around 36 weeks of pregnancy is a good time to do this, because your breasts will have done most of

Tips on buying bras for breastfeeding

- Make sure the bra fits well, with enough space in the cups to allow for some expansion when your breasts are full.
- If you're buying a bra near the end of your pregnancy, make sure you're not using the tightest fastening already.
- Avoid styles with underwiring or tight edges that could press into your breasts and squash some of the ducts.
- Go for cups that open fully, so your baby's access to your breast isn't restricted.
- Wide straps are more comfortable than narrow ones if your breasts are heavy.
- If possible, choose a style that's easy to unfasten and re-fasten with one hand.
- Choose cotton bras; synthetic fabrics will prevent your skin from breathing.
- Expect to need at least three bras, to cope with leaks (especially in the early weeks).

their growing but your rib cage won't yet have expanded fully, so the bra should fit well when you no longer have a bump. Badly fitting bras can squash the milk ducts, and may cause them to become blocked.

Wearing a bra at night will allow you to wear breast pads if leaking is a problem. Night-time feeding bras are usually light and stretchy with no hook fastenings at the back, making them comfortable to sleep in.

Do I need special clothes?

There are special clothes you can buy for breastfeeding, such as tops with hidden openings and breastfeeding shawls, but there's really no need to kit yourself out with these unless you want to. Ordinary loose-fitting tops can usually be lifted up with one hand without exposing too much flesh, enabling feeding to be discreet if it needs to be. (Tight-fitting tops can encourage leaking and tend to show off breast pads.)

If you're worried about displaying your post-pregnancy 'jelly-belly' when you lift your top, you may want to buy a breastfeeding vest or nursing top which has a second, shorter layer of fabric underneath the main T-shirt. This layer stays in place over your tummy when the outer bit is raised. Alternatively, you can create something similar by wearing a low-cut vest underneath a loose top – just pull the loose top up and the vest down for feeding. Another option is to wear maternity trousers or leggings, with a high waistband that comes up to your breasts, covering your stomach.

If you want to cover up when you are feeding outside the home, a simple muslin square over your shoulder, or a loose-fitting cardigan or scarf pulled around you, may be the easiest solution. Whatever you decide, after a little practice you'll probably find you can breastfeed without anyone knowing what you're doing.

What equipment do I need?

If you're planning to breastfeed you don't really need many of the baby-feeding products aimed at expectant parents. Although most women find breast pads and muslins useful it's probably best to wait until your baby arrives before buying other things.

If you're going back to work you may want bottles and perhaps a breast pump, but you won't need them straight away – and if you wait until you're ready to express, you may get a better feel for which models will suit your needs. Many women find they don't need to express milk, or that it's just as quick – and more effective – by hand. You may think you're bound to need dummies but they can seriously interfere with breastfeeding in the early days (see pages 39 and 75), so are best avoided for at least the first few weeks.

Some mothers find breastfeeding pillows useful but one size doesn't fit all, and using a pillow in the early days may prevent you and your baby finding the most comfortable position for feeding (see page 47). Experimenting with a normal bedroom pillow, or with different types of breastfeeding pillows (maybe at a breastfeeding group or in the shop) once your baby is born will help you decide, but many mothers find that a scrunched-up cardigan or baby blanket is more flexible and easier to carry around.

A sling (or baby carrier) is probably one of the most useful pieces of baby equipment but it's worth waiting until your baby arrives to buy one. That way you can experiment with friends' slings or those in shops to find out which style works best for you – especially if you want to be able to feed your baby while you're 'wearing' him.

'I love the freedom breastfeeding gives me compared to bottle feeding. I'll just put him in a sling, shove a nappy, spare babygro and a muslin into a little bag and that's all we need. My friends doing formula always seem so weighed down with stuff.'

Nicky, mother of Charlie, five months

Key points

- Almost all women can breastfeed.

- Breastfeeding can help your baby resist infections and diseases throughout his life. Not breastfeeding carries health risks for your baby, and for you.

- The more you breastfeed, and the longer you do it for, the greater the health protection for you and your baby.

- Breastfeeding isn't just about nutrition – it can make parenting easier.

- There is a lot of out-dated and confusing advice around breastfeeding. Take time to learn how breastfeeding works and why letting your baby lead the way makes sense.

- Make sure your partner and family understand about breastfeeding, too, so that they can support you.

- All sizes and shapes of breasts work for breastfeeding. You don't need to do anything special to get yours ready.

- Breastfeeding bras should be fitted when you are around 36 weeks pregnant. Avoid underwires and non-cotton fabrics.

- It's usually better to buy pumps and bottles once you know what will suit you and your baby – you may not need them at all.

- Trying out different slings and pillows once your baby is born is the best way to work out what you need.

2

How milk production works

Baby-led breastfeeding means helping your breasts to work naturally. This means getting milk production kick-started in the first two weeks and always letting your baby feed whenever she wants, for as long as she wants. Feeding this way will ensure that she gets the nourishment she needs and that your milk supply keeps pace with her changing appetite.

The early days and weeks after the birth are enormously important for breastfeeding. What happens during this time can make a big difference to how much milk you are able to produce later on. This chapter explains how breastmilk is made and how frequent feeding and keeping your baby close will help you make as much as your baby needs for as long as she needs it.

What your breasts look like inside

To understand how to get the best from your breasts, it helps to understand their structure. Whatever your breasts look like from the outside, the inside is pretty much the same for all women – except for the amount of fat. Large breasts contain more fatty tissue than smaller ones, not more milk-making tissue – so size doesn't matter when it comes to breastfeeding.

Here's what your breasts look like inside:

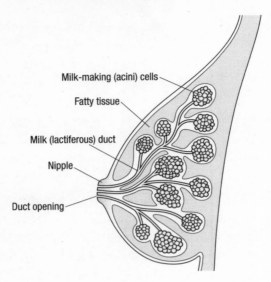

Milk-making (acini) cells

Fatty tissue

Milk (lactiferous) duct

Nipple

Duct opening

Under a microscope, the milk-making tissue looks a bit like bunches of grapes. Each 'grape', or alveolus, is a cluster of milk-making cells called acini cells. The acini cells make milk by taking the ingredients for breastmilk from your bloodstream and combining them in the right proportions. The 'stalks' are the tubes, or lactiferous ducts, that carry the milk out of the breast via the nipple.

Getting your breasts to make milk

During pregnancy, milk production is minimal, with the breasts producing small amounts of colostrum only. This changes immediately the placenta is delivered. When a newborn baby is placed on her mother's front, with their skin touching ('skin to skin'), she will instinctively move her head and wriggle around to find the breast. This nuzzling triggers the release of a hormone called prolactin into the mother's bloodstream. Prolactin is detected by a sensitive area on each milk-making cell and it has the effect of priming them, or switching them on. **Skin-to-skin contact between mother and baby is a crucial factor in switching on milk production – even if the baby doesn't actually feed straight away.**

The brain also has sensitive areas that detect prolactin. When these are stimulated they make the mother want to protect her baby and hold her close. This combination of *your* instinct to keep your baby safe and her instinct to find your breast makes sure she has access to the food she needs.

If lots of milk-making cells are switched on, your breasts will be able to respond effectively and quickly whenever your baby needs more milk. This means you'll have plenty of milk as she grows, and be able to meet her need for extra quantities when she has an appetite spurt (also known as a growth spurt or hunger spurt) or is teething or ill. A milk-making cell that is properly switched on soon after birth will keep producing milk for as long as it's needed but any cells that haven't been fully primed will start to shut down – and they can't be re-activated until the next pregnancy. Breasts which have only a few cells switched on are set up for minimum milk production only, so they won't be able to respond when the baby needs extra milk.

Holding your baby skin to skin as soon as she's born, and continuing to hold her and allow her to feed as much as you can in the first two weeks will help you to switch on the maximum number of milk-making cells, so that you can continue to make as much milk as she needs for as long as you want. And if you have two babies there'll be twice the stimulation, so twice as much switching on.

If you and your baby can't be together during the early weeks (if one of you is ill, for example), getting milk production up and running will be more challenging, but it's certainly not impossible. See page 187 for information on how to make sure your breasts get switched on even if your baby isn't able to help. On page 217 there's information on how to start breastfeeding later, even if you've started your baby on formula.

The role of the 'love' hormone

When a baby and her mother are close to each other another important hormone, oxytocin, is released into the mother's bloodstream. Oxytocin is often referred to as the love hormone. It's responsible for:

- Making you fall in love.
- Helping you to get pregnant (by making you feel relaxed so you lie down after an orgasm).
- Making your womb contract during labour (and afterwards).
- Helping you to fall in love (or 'bond') with your newborn baby.
- Making your milk available to your baby.

When a baby suckles at her mother's breast, huge bursts of oxytocin are triggered, making the little muscles that surround the milk-making cells and the ducts contract. This squeezes the milk down the ducts and is called the let-down reflex, or the milk ejection reflex. If the reflex is very strong, milk may leak (or even squirt) out of the nipples (see photo number 6). **It's a combination of this let-down reflex and the squeezing action of the baby's tongue (see page 32) that allows her to get milk.** In the first week or so, the let-down reflex is a bit erratic and it may not happen for a minute or two after the baby starts suckling. However, it soon settles down so that it coincides with the beginning of each feed.

Some women feel their let-down reflex as a pinching or tingling sensation inside their breasts. Many also say that it gives them a nice woozy feeling, helping them to relax and focus on their baby. Some describe it as being like the relaxed

BREASTFEEDING CAN MAKE YOU SLEEPY

Breastfeeding is no more tiring than bottle feeding but the effects of oxytocin can make you want to curl up and snooze. This is useful at night but it may be a bit unexpected during the day. You can either go with the flow, and have a nap while your baby sleeps (which is really what your body is telling you to do), or shake off the sleepy feeling by getting up and moving around.

feeling they get after an orgasm (not surprising really, when the same hormone is responsible for both). So oxytocin not only helps mothers to feed their babies but it makes caring for your baby more pleasurable and less stressful as well.

In the early days women often feel after-pains (a bit like period pains) when their let-down reflex happens. This is oxytocin making the womb contract, helping it to get back to its non-pregnant size and reducing blood loss. (Mothers who are not breastfeeding get after-pains, too – but not necessarily when they're feeding their baby.) This connection between oxytocin, the womb and the breasts can sometimes work when you don't expect it – for example, making your breasts tingle, and even leak, when you're making love.

Production on demand – how it works

A breastfeeding mother's breasts are never truly empty; breastmilk is being made constantly, so there is always some-thing there for the baby, even when she has just fed. However, the rate at which milk is made varies. If the breast is full or if there are long gaps between feeds, production slows down; if the baby feeds more often or drains the breast more effec-tively, milk making speeds up.

All of this happens because breastmilk contains something called the Feedback Inhibitor of Lactation – or FIL, for short. The amount of FIL is dependent on the amount of milk in the breast and its function is to reduce production when it seems the milk isn't needed. So if your baby is feeding infrequently, or has had a longer than usual gap between feeds, your milk-making cells will respond by slowing down. But if she feeds frequently, your breasts will carry on producing milk at a steady rate. Feeding two or more babies means the breasts are almost never allowed to get full, so production is maintained at a high rate. More feeding means more milk.

After the first few weeks it's FIL and the amount of milk in your breasts (rather than simply how often your baby feeds) that controls how quickly more is made. **If your baby isn't removing milk effectively when she feeds, your milk production will slow down even if she goes to the breast frequently.** See Chapter 6 for information on making sure her feeding is effective.

The FIL mechanism works separately in each breast. This means each breast will only make as much milk as it is asked to make. Some babies feed more on one breast than the other, or even feed exclusively from one breast. When this happens FIL makes sure that the other breast doesn't keep producing milk that isn't needed (and which would make the mother uncomfortable on that side). Much later, when breastfeeding is coming to an end, it's FIL that helps milk production to wind down gradually and comfortably.

The way FIL works means that, as long as your milk-making cells have been primed, you can increase or decrease milk production on demand. If your baby needs more milk, feeding her more frequently will put in the order for extra to be made. There will be a delay of a few feeds but you'll soon notice production increasing. The same thing applies in reverse: if feeds get further apart, production slows down – but again, it will take your breasts a few feeds to adjust. It's all about telling your breasts what's needed.

How to make sure your baby gets enough milk

The best way to be sure your baby gets all the milk she needs is to:

- Let her feed whenever she wants.
- Let her feed for as long as she wants at each feed.
- When she finishes feeding on the first breast, *offer* her the second (but don't worry if she turns it down).

This is the essence of baby-led breastfeeding. Feeding this way will ensure that your baby gets the nourishment she needs and that your milk production keeps pace with her changing appetite. It is also more likely to lead to easy, pain-free feeding than following a pre-determined schedule or routine.

How breastmilk changes to meet your baby's needs

Breastmilk changes during the course of a single feed and throughout the day. It also changes as the baby gets older, to meet her growing needs.

The first milk

The first milk produced by your breasts is called colostrum. It's usually yellowish and sticky – a bit like clear honey. Colostrum is a concentrated version of breastmilk. It's packed with important nutrients and antibodies to nourish your baby and protect her from infection and it comes in small quantities, for some very good reasons.

Once she's born your baby needs to learn how to co-ordinate sucking and swallowing with breathing; colostrum allows her a couple of days to practise this new skill before she has to cope with larger volumes of milk. At the same time it allows her kidneys to adapt gently to life outside the womb, and her stomach – which is tiny at birth – to expand and adjust gradually to taking in more milk.

Over the first four or five days, your milk will become less concentrated as other ingredients (especially water) become part of the recipe. If your baby is allowed to feed frequently, she'll gradually be able to manage larger feeds as the volume of milk increases. But if she doesn't feed often, she may well find the amount of milk – and the strong flow – difficult to cope with. There's also a good chance that your breasts will become overfull, leading to engorgement (see page 235). Offering your baby the chance to feed when you feel your breasts becoming full will help to prevent discomfort for you, as well as keeping the flow manageable for her.

It used to be thought that colostrum only lasted for three days – until the 'real milk' came in. In fact, pretty much all the ingredients of colostrum, including the antibodies that protect against disease, continue to be made. Colostrum is special because it is so concentrated, which is what a newborn baby needs. Later milk is less concentrated but is just as nutritious and protective as colostrum.

MY BREASTMILK IS ORANGE!

The colour of breastmilk changes over the first few days, usually becoming creamy-white or white. A small amount of blood in the milk (caused by the normal increase in blood flow to the breasts in the first week or so) can turn it pink or orange. This is known as 'rusty pipe syndrome'. Later, other colours are possible, too: some mothers say their milk looks bluish, while others find that eating a lot of leafy vegetables gives their milk a green tinge. All of these variations are normal (but see page 231 for more on blood in breastmilk).

Breastmilk changes during a feed

Once the colostrum-only stage is over, the composition of your milk will change gradually during each feed. The first few mouthfuls from each breast are quite watery – a sort of drink or soup course – then the amount of fat begins to increase, with the milk getting progressively more fatty through the main course to the dessert. The more watery milk is sometimes referred to as 'foremilk' and the fatty milk as 'hindmilk' but these terms are misleading. There aren't two sorts of milk and there isn't a single point during the feed when the milk changes from one type to the other. It just gets gradually creamier (and higher in calories) with every mouthful.

Breastmilk changes over a day

Your breastmilk will vary slightly over the course of a day. For example, when your baby has just finished feeding, the milk remaining in that breast will be very fatty, whereas half an hour later it will be more watery again. The rate of milk production will also vary; most mothers say they produce more milk in the morning than in the evening.

Some research suggests that milk produced in the evening is higher in fat than that produced earlier in the day and that night-time milk contains a natural sleep-inducing chemical that calms babies and helps them to fall asleep. Whether or not this is true, breastfeeding at night has a soothing effect on both mother and baby (see page 25).

Breastmilk changes as your baby gets older

Your breastmilk will continue to change as your baby gets older. Your breasts will adjust the ingredients very slightly all the time, in line with her growing needs, and the antibody content will vary according to the infections your body detects around you (see *Amazing antibodies*, page 7). Then, as breastfeeding gradually winds down, your milk will become more like colostrum again. This is because a child who isn't feeding often but is out in the big wide world, exposed to lots of germs, needs concentrated shots of protective antibodies, just as she did when she was newborn.

Your baby knows what she needs

Breastmilk can be food or drink – or both. Sometimes your baby will want a quick drink, so she'll just have a few mouthfuls of milk from one breast. If she's really thirsty she may come off the first breast and want a couple of sucks from the second as well. On another occasion she'll want a 'three-course meal' from one breast and a 'drink' from the second – or she may decide to stay on the second breast for longer, so that she gets double helpings of all three courses. Sometimes she'll even want to go back to the first breast again! All of this is quite normal.

Babies don't need any other drinks, even in hot weather. In fact, giving babies even small drinks of water can fill their tummies and dull their appetite for milk, reducing their resistance to illness and possibly limiting their weight gain. The breasts reset themselves very quickly between feeds in terms of the fat/water balance, so a new feed will always be thirst-quenching. **Your baby is the only one who knows what she needs – you can trust her to get the right balance of food and fluid when she feeds.**

Key points

- Skin-to-skin contact with your baby and frequent feeding 'switch on' your milk-making cells.

- The more feeding you do early on, the more milk you can make long term. Milk production can then be stepped up or down later, according to your baby's needs.

- When your baby suckles, oxytocin – the 'love hormone' – triggers your let-down reflex, which sends your milk down the ducts towards the nipple.

- Feeding on demand ensures you keep making plenty of milk. If you let your breasts get too full, milk production will slow down.

- Breastmilk starts off as colostrum, which is packed full of nutrients and protective ingredients. It becomes less concentrated over the first few days as the amount increases.

- Breastmilk can be food or drink, or both. It gradually changes throughout a feed, from watery (thirst-quenching) to creamy (full of calories).

- Breastfeeding works best when it's baby-led.

3

How to breastfeed

Babies have a natural instinct for breastfeeding and don't need to be taught what to do. However, they do need the opportunity to work out how to do it, and they need plenty of practice in the beginning if they're to get good at it quickly. Baby-led breastfeeding is about trusting your baby's abilities and allowing plenty of time for him to learn. It's about holding him in a way that makes it easy for him to feed, rather than in a particular position, and being aware of things that could make breastfeeding more difficult for him. Following his lead means he will get the milk he needs, and you will avoid many common problems.

This chapter explains how your baby attaches to the breast to feed, what he has to do to get milk out of your breast and what you can do to help him become skilled at breastfeeding.

The secret of pain-free feeding – attachment

The secret to effective, pain-free breastfeeding lies in the attachment between the baby's mouth and the breast. To get lots of milk, your baby's mouth needs to be full of breast, so he can squeeze the milk from the ducts easily. And to feed without hurting you, he needs to have your nipple right at the back of his mouth, where it can't be damaged.

To get the milk out your baby will use his tongue and lower jaw in a combination of 'yawning' and squeezing. He'll open his mouth wide (like the baby in photo number 23), scoop up a large mouthful of breast and nipple, and make a secure seal with his lips. Then he'll:

- Drop his lower jaw in a yawning movement (without breaking the seal), to allow the ducts to fill with milk.
- Raise his jaw again, trapping some of the milk in the ducts.
- Use his tongue to press the breast against the roof of his mouth, squeezing the trapped milk out of the nipple into the back of his mouth.
- Swallow the milk.

He'll repeat this cycle over and over, in a rhythmic way while he's feeding.

If your baby has hold of just the nipple and a small amount of breast:

- He'll lose his grip easily when he tries to drop his lower jaw.
- There won't be much milk available for him to squeeze out.
- Your nipple will be pinched against his hard palate.
- He'll have to suck hard to keep the nipple in his mouth.
- He'll get tired long before he's had a satisfying feed.
- Your breast won't be effectively drained and your nipple may get damaged.

The result could be, for you:

- sore nipples
- engorgement
- mastitis
- a slowing down of milk production.

And for your baby:

- frustration
- exhaustion
- constant hunger
- slow weight gain.

Sometimes a baby can seem to be feeding well at the beginning of a feed, when the mother's let-down reflex (see page 24) is at its strongest. But once the reflex subsides and the milk flow slows down, if he isn't effectively attached he won't be able to get big mouthfuls of milk and he'll become frustrated or tired. If this is repeated at every feed, his mother's

---

Breastfeeding is different from bottle feeding

Many people assume that breastfeeding is like drinking from a bottle with a teat but it's very different. Here's why:

Put the end of your thumb into your mouth and give it a few sucks. Notice how much of your tongue is in contact with your thumb and how it moves against it. This is like bottle feeding. Now put your thumb right in – up to the second joint – and suck it again. This is like breastfeeding.

When your thumb is deep inside your mouth, much more of your tongue is in contact with it, so you can use your tongue to squeeze it against the roof of your mouth. The tip of your thumb is free, up by your soft palate (the squashy bit at the back) where there's more space. And you don't have to keep sucking to hold on to it.

This is why your nipple needs to be in the back of your baby's mouth when he breastfeeds. If he tries to feed as if he is sucking from a bottle, your nipple will be squashed, it will be harder for him to keep it in his mouth and he won't get enough milk. He needs a good mouthful of breast *plus* nipple to feed effectively.

breasts will have more milk left in them than they should, and they'll get the message that less is needed.

Your baby knows how to breastfeed

Babies have a strong instinct to breastfeed. They are born wanting to find the breast and they go through a very distinctive pattern of behaviour to help them do this (see page 56). Recognising your baby's instincts – and allowing him to use them – will give him the best chance of breast-feeding effectively.

When they are near the breast, babies bob their heads around and use their hands in a kneading action to orientate themselves and work out how best to approach the nipple. This behaviour is a crucial part of the feed because it allows the baby to get to the breast and position himself so that he can attach easily. It will happen more quickly as your baby gets more skilled but it's important that he isn't disturbed or hurried if he seems to be taking his time in the first few weeks.

When he can feel or smell that he is near his mother's nipple, a baby will naturally start to open his mouth and stretch his tongue forwards. This is known as 'rooting' and it's part of his preparation for scooping up the breast to feed. **Once he's worked out where the nipple is, he'll tip his head back. This helps him to open his mouth really wide and come to the breast chin first.** It also means that, if the nipple was roughly level with his nose beforehand, it will now be near his top lip and pointing towards the roof of his mouth. All of this helps him to get a really good mouthful of breast, with the nipple touching his soft palate.

Working with your baby – 'latching on'

The moment when a baby attaches to his mother's breast is sometimes known as 'latching on'. It's a crucial part of breastfeeding but it usually happens in less time than it's taken you to read these two sentences. One minute your baby is bouncing his head against your breast and the next he's taking his first gulp. Blink and you'll miss it. What happens during these few seconds – and whether or not your baby attaches successfully – depends on whether his mouth and your breast can make contact easily.

Getting the angle right

Your baby needs to scoop up your breast with the nipple pointing towards the roof of his mouth, rather than straight on, because otherwise his tongue will get in the way. The space for your breast is in the *upper* part of his mouth, not the middle. (If you put your finger into your own mouth, first centrally and then pointing upwards, you'll feel how high up the space is.) If your nipple goes into your baby's mouth centrally, he won't be able to draw it deep inside, so he won't get much milk (and he may make you sore). Photos number 15 to 17 show a baby scooping up the breast at just the right angle.

Mothers are sometimes told they need to make sure *all* the areola is in their baby's mouth when he feeds. This isn't true. The areola is just a part of your skin and most areolas are too large to fit inside a baby's mouth. **What is important is that, if your areola is an even shape, with the nipple in the middle of it, when your baby is feeding, you should be able to see more of your areola above his top lip than below his bottom lip** (as in photo number 18).

In order to achieve this angle, your baby needs to tip his head back and come to the breast with his chin leading. He will do this instinctively, provided nothing stops him. However, any sort of pressure on his head – even just a finger – will prevent him from tilting his head back and will push his nose (rather than his chin) into your breast. Not only will this make it difficult for him to attach and feed, it may also make him cross and lead to him 'fighting' at the breast. Depending on his position, you may need to support your baby's neck and shoulders – but try to avoid holding his head, so that he can tip it back easily (see *How do I hold my baby for feeding?*, page 41).

Getting the timing right

If you are lying back with your baby on top of you, gravity will help him to attach, so you won't need to do very much at all. He'll attach himself when he's ready – as the baby in photos 20 to 24 demonstrates. If you're holding him in another position, you'll need to be ready to bring him closer to your breast at just the right moment. This means moving him quickly towards you (*not* pushing your breast towards him), when his mouth is at its widest. Babies don't tend to hold their mouths open for very long so the best moment for latching on only lasts a second. If you miss it, just ease your baby away and start again.

If your baby's first attempt to attach doesn't result in a large mouthful of breast, he'll probably let go and try again, opening his mouth a little wider this time. However, some babies are reluctant to open their mouths really wide, usually because they haven't learnt that this is what they need to do. If your baby attaches without scooping up a good mouthful of breast he probably won't get much milk and he is likely to make you sore.

If your baby doesn't seem to want to open his mouth wide, express a drop of milk so he can smell it on your nipple, or touch it to his lips so he can taste it. If this doesn't tempt him, rub his nose gently against your nipple and then move him away. A brief, light touch, repeated several times, will be more effective than simply holding him with his nose against your breast. Keep 'teasing' him like this – without letting him attach – until he opens his mouth really wide.

THAT OUCH! MOMENT

You may experience an 'ouch' moment at the beginning of feeds in the first few days, while you and your baby are getting your positioning and timing sorted out. This shouldn't last more than about 10 seconds. If it does, just take him off your breast and start again. (Slip a finger into the corner of his mouth to break the suction before easing him away gently, so that you don't damage your nipple.)

Sometimes babies become agitated and end up sucking their fists instead of the breast, as though they're confused about what they should be doing. This is normal behaviour. Sucking has a soothing effect, so sucking his fists helps a fretful baby to calm down. And moving his hand between the breast and his mouth also helps him to find exactly where the nipple is. Focusing on relaxing *yourself* and talking gently to your baby will help him to relax and work out what he needs to do.

What makes latching on difficult?

The most likely reason why babies find it difficult to attach (or latch on) to the breast is that they are not being held in the most helpful way (see page 41 for information on holding your baby for feeding). Another common reason is that the breast is overfull, making it difficult to scoop up. In this case hand expressing a little milk (see page 86) will soften your breast and make it easier for your baby to manage.

Overfull breasts are often the result of a long gap between feeds – and a long gap can mean a very hungry baby. Being over-hungry is stressful and this can make it difficult for the baby to relax and let his instincts guide him (especially if he has been crying) so he struggles to attach effectively. This makes the baby more stressed and can easily lead to a vicious cycle, where feeding is painful for the mother and frustrating for them both.

Feeding whenever your baby wants to, and offering him a feed as soon as you notice your breasts feeling full – even if he's asleep – should prevent him getting too hungry *and* keep your breasts from becoming uncomfortable. It will also give him plenty of opportunity to fine-tune his technique.

Long or very wide nipples can occasionally make latching on difficult because they trick the baby into starting to suck before he's scooped up enough of the breast. If your baby is struggling to get a big enough mouthful because you have large nipples, you may be able to help him by gently pressing your thumb into your breast *just above your baby's nose* to tilt the nipple up slightly as you offer it to him, then let it unfold into his mouth. This will help him to scoop up more than just the nipple. It will also exaggerate the angle at which the nipple points inside his mouth, helping him to draw it in deeply before he starts sucking.

A baby who has a tongue tie (see box, below) may also find latching on difficult.

Bottles and dummies can interfere

A baby doesn't need to scoop up a teat (or dummy). In fact, he only needs to open his mouth a little way and someone will pop it in for him. Many babies who have been given a teat or a dummy while they are learning to breastfeed subsequently make only half-hearted attempts to open their mouth, or they latch on to the nipple alone, instead of the breast. This doesn't *always* happen but it's impossible to predict which babies will react like this, so if you do plan to introduce a teat, it's best to avoid it for a few weeks until your baby has got the hang of breastfeeding (see *Getting breastfeeding 'established'*, page 108).

WHAT IS A TONGUE TIE?

In babies with tongue tie the frenulum, which joins the tongue to the floor of the mouth, extends farther forward than usual. This extra membrane restricts the movement of the tongue and prevents the baby from scooping up and compressing the breast effectively. He may slip off the breast easily, feed very briefly and ask to feed again after only a few minutes. He's also likely to get frustrated and tired at the breast – and his mother may develop sore nipples. A tongue tie can make bottle feeding difficult, too.

A tongue tie is sometimes easy to see, because the tip of the baby's tongue makes a heart shape when he tries to stretch it forward, but it isn't always obvious. Some babies who appear to have a tongue tie can breastfeed without a problem. Others can be helped to attach effectively if the mother tilts her nipple upwards (by pressing gently with her thumb opposite the baby's nose) as her baby scoops up the breast. Feeding positions where the baby is more upright can also help (see below).

It's important that tongue tie is diagnosed early, so that the mother and baby can get help with breastfeeding. Some babies need their frenulum to be cut or 'divided', which is usually quick and painless, with the baby being handed straight to his mother afterwards for a feed. (Older babies are inclined to wriggle, so they may need an anaesthetic.) If your baby seems to be finding breastfeeding difficult, contact someone with expertise in breastfeeding (see *Where can I get help?*, page 106) as soon as you can.

Nipple shields rarely help

Nipple shields are sometimes recommended for mothers whose nipples are flat or inverted, or when babies are having difficulties attaching to the breast. These soft silicone devices are worn over the nipple and areola during breastfeeding.

However, just like a teat, they can be poked into a baby's mouth and can make it *appear* as though the baby is feeding well. In reality, many babies will struggle to accommodate a shield *and* scoop up the amount of breast they need to feed effectively. And they will learn to expect the shield, meaning it can be difficult, later, to persuade them to feed without it.

Nipple shields may also cut down the amount of stimulation the breasts get while the baby is feeding (leading to reduced milk production). Some mothers who have a tendency to produce more milk than their baby needs (see page 212) *may* be able to feed with a nipple shield long term but for most women they are best avoided.

How do I hold my baby for feeding?

A lot of books and leaflets about breastfeeding give detailed instructions involving special chairs, pillows, footstools and ways to hold the baby. All of this can make breastfeeding

Your body shape makes a difference

Your body shape will influence the way you need to hold your baby for feeding. Look in a mirror: notice how your breasts hang and which way your nipples point (sometimes referred to as your 'angle of dangle'!). A mother with small, pert breasts will need to hold her baby much higher up her body than a mother whose breasts are large and pendulous, with downward-pointing nipples, and her baby will need to face her in a slightly different way. It's quite likely, too, that your right breast hangs slightly differently from the left one, so be prepared to adjust the way you hold your baby when he swaps sides. There's no standard breastfeeding position – you'll soon find what works for you and your baby.

much more complicated than it needs to be. Time spent getting yourself and your baby into exactly the 'right' position for feeding is likely to make him frustrated and unable to latch on easily, so feeding becomes unnecessarily stressful for both of you.

Every woman is built in a unique way. Your body proportions, breasts and nipples are different from other women's. And, of course, each baby is different too. All these things affect how you will hold your baby for feeding – and they mean that it's difficult for anyone to predict exactly what you'll need to do without knowing a bit about you and your baby.

It's your baby's position that matters

The way you sit, stand or lie at the start of a breastfeed doesn't really matter, provided you're reasonably comfortable – what matters is how *your baby* is positioned. This is what will determine whether or not he can breastfeed effectively, without causing you pain. Once he's feeding, you can move around and adjust your own position (see page 47), if you need to.

There are lots of different ways to hold your baby for breastfeeding and babies (especially older ones) can feed in all sorts of positions, as photos 25 to 34 show. But for a position to work it must allow your baby to use his hands to help

DRINKING COMFORTABLY

To understand how your baby's position matters, try drinking a glass of water with your head turned sideways. Or ask someone to put their hand on the back of your head, to stop you tipping it back while you drink. How easy is it for you to open your mouth, tip your glass and swallow if your neck is twisted or you can't tip your head back? It's no different for your baby when he's trying to breastfeed.

Essentials for helping your baby to feed

For your newborn baby to be able to attach and feed effectively, he needs to be:

- close to you, with
- as much of his body in contact with yours as possible (check for gaps – his chest and hips should be touching you; pull his bottom in close)
- his whole body in line (i.e. with his knees facing the same way as his nose)
- his body weight supported (neck, shoulders and hips)
- his head and arms free to move, and
- his nose lined up with your nipple ('nose to nipple').

These factors are important, however you hold your baby for feeding; they happen automatically in some feeding positions but can easily be overlooked in others.

him, to tilt his head back easily, and to scoop up your breast with your nipple pointing towards the roof of his mouth.

Lying back can be a good way to feed

One of the easiest positions for a baby to learn to feed in is lying on his tummy, with his mother half sitting and half lying, supported by pillows or cushions (see photos number 20, 21, 25 and 34). This is sometimes known as the 'laid-back' or Biological Nurturing™ position. This position is easy for your baby because:

- He is close to your breast, so he doesn't have to stretch (and you aren't tempted to lean forwards and give yourself backache).

- Your breast is underneath him, so gravity helps him to attach and to stay attached (rather than pulling him away, as it would do if you were more upright).
- He is facing your breast, so he doesn't have to twist awkwardly.
- He can lift and turn his head freely, using his arms to help him balance.
- He can change his position to bring his nose into line with your nipple (so that when he tilts his head back the nipple will be aiming at the roof of his mouth).
- His whole body is in contact with you, so he feels safe.
- You don't have to support his weight with your arms.
- You don't have to judge when he is ready to attach or help him by bringing him to your breast at the right moment.
- You can trust him to position himself, rather than feeling that you have to get everything 'right'.

The first breastfeed happens like this for many babies (see Chapter 4), and it's the position that will make best use of your baby's feeding instincts when he is new. Many mothers also find it easier because all they have to do is to stop their baby falling sideways – which makes it especially useful for feeding twins. (You'll need to adapt it slightly after a Caesarean section, though – see page 63.)

Feeding this way allows your baby more control than being held in your arms and gives him a better chance of learning how to feed effectively. This will make it easier for him to adapt to other feeding positions later. However, feeding like this doesn't need to be limited to when your baby is young or while he is learning to feed – you can feed a child of any age this way. It's especially useful in the evenings, when many babies want to have lots of feeds close together, because it allows you to simply lie back on the sofa with your feet up while your baby 'helps himself'.

'It took me months before I realised I didn't have to feed my baby cradled in my arms. A friend told me she fed lying down – I couldn't believe it! So then I fed like that a lot – even during the day, sometimes on my side and sometimes with me on my back on pillows and the baby on my chest. And when Rachael was big enough, I'd sit on a chair and she'd just have a quick feed standing up!'

Michelle, mother of Rachael, four years

There are no set positions for feeding

Although lying back to feed is great for learning, there will be situations when another position will be more convenient, so it's worth exploring a few options. Lots of books describe specific positions for breastfeeding but, provided it works for you and your baby, in reality anything goes. Whether he's wrapped across your front, tucked under your arm, or lying next to you on a bed, the same basic principles apply (see *Essentials for helping your baby to feed,* page 43). If what you've chosen is helpful for him he'll be able to attach to the breast and feed easily. If it's *unhelpful* he may struggle to get a good mouthful or find it difficult to suck or swallow.

It's easy to be tempted to start off by cradling your baby with his head resting in the crook of your elbow. This position is fine for bottle feeding but it doesn't work for breastfeeding. It won't allow your baby to reach the breast comfortably (without twisting), tip his head back or swallow

---

TIP

If you're supporting your baby's neck and shoulders with your hand, watch that your fingertips and thumb don't creep up the edges of his ears. If they do he won't be able to tip his head back and latch on at the right angle.

easily. If you want to cradle your baby in your arms to feed, make sure he's facing your nipple and rest his neck on your forearm instead.

There's no need to aim to have eye contact with your baby while he's feeding. Babies enjoy feeding in a variety of positions – and many feed with their eyes closed. You and your baby will be communicating throughout every feed through touch and smell so eye contact isn't necessary.

As you experiment with a few different positions, you'll find one or two that are favourites for you and your baby, but they may not always turn out the way you expected. Don't be surprised to find that:

- When you hold your baby across your front to feed from one breast, most of his body is over by your other breast (as in photos number 28 and 32).
- When you hold your baby under your arm to feed (sometimes called the 'rugby' hold, see photos number

BREATHING WHILE FEEDING

There's normally no need to hold your breast away from your baby's nose while he feeds. If he's been allowed to come to the breast 'nose to nipple', and to tip his head back and attach with his chin leading, his nostrils will be free. If a cushion, or tight clothing, is pushing the breast into your baby's nose, it's better to move what's causing the problem than to press your finger into your breast.

If your baby's nose is buried in your breast it's unlikely his chin will be pressed into it, which means he hasn't got a good mouthful. Holding the breast away from his nose may allow him to breathe but it won't enable him to feed effectively. It may also prevent some of your ducts from draining properly. He needs to be helped to come off the breast and start again.

26 and 33), most of his body is behind you. (You may need to make sure he isn't pushing himself too far forward with his feet.)

- When you lie down on your side to feed (see photo number 31), your baby's shoulders are well below your breast. (You may need to straighten your legs until he is attached and feeding, so that he doesn't use your thighs to push himself upwards.)

It's worth finding a few different positions that you and your baby like and to vary the way you hold him occasionally, just to help make sure that milk is removed from all parts of your breasts. This will help to prevent you developing blocked ducts (see page 237).

Getting comfortable once your baby is feeding

As long as you are holding your baby in a way that allows him to breastfeed easily, how you position yourself is a personal thing. The best approach is to focus on *your baby's* needs first and work out what else *you* might need once he's feeding. This will save a lot of time and make life easier for both of you. Don't assume you'll need a pillow to support him – struggling to position your baby *and* a pillow can make things more difficult.

'When I fed the twins together I'd often sit cross-legged so I could move my knees to position each baby individually.'

Siobhan, mother of Connor, four years, Orla and Sophie, two years

Once your baby has latched on and started to feed, think about whether you need to change your position slightly. Wriggle around a bit to get comfortable. If you need to move (for instance, to sit more upright or lean back), hold your baby firmly against your body so that you take him with you as you adjust your position. Provided he was able to latch on easily, and you brought him to your breast rather than moving your breast towards him, his attachment will usually be secure enough to allow you to move without him becoming dislodged. You may want to stuff a cushion, baby blanket, cardigan or towel under your elbow (to help you support your baby's weight) or in the small of your back. You are the best judge of what needs to be where, so don't be afraid to experiment.

'Feeding Joe was painful but I'd be too nervous to move him, so I would just put up with it. But with Bella, I take her off if it's not right and once she's on okay I move round to make sure we are both comfortable. I'm much more relaxed and we haven't had any problems so far.'

Jackie, mother of Joe, three years, and Bella, six weeks

Do I need to hold my breast?

There's no need to grip your breast while your baby is feeding. He comes to your breast, not the other way around, so it's not necessary to lift your breast up, point it in a certain direction or try to put the nipple in your baby's mouth for him. Distorting the breast's natural shape can interfere with the instincts that help a baby to breastfeed. And having your fingers pressing into your breast during a feed may prevent your milk flowing properly.

You may find it helpful to steady your breast while your baby is attaching but, unless it's very heavy, you should be able to release it once he's attached. Some mothers with large breasts find they can see what they're doing more easily if they support their breast underneath and use their thumb to flatten the top slightly, just until their baby is attached. If you're worried that letting go of your breast will make your baby lose his grip, experiment with moving him down a little first, so that the weight of the breast doesn't pull it away from him.

If you have very heavy breasts, you may find you are more comfortable if you support the weight of your breast throughout the feed. You can use your hand to do it, but that will tend to push your baby away from you and may make feeding difficult for him. It might help to use your other hand to support him so that your breast-supporting hand is out of his way, as in photo number 32 (sometimes known as the cross-cradle position). If you find that taking the weight of your breast makes your arm ache you may find it easier to put a small rolled-up flannel or muslin cloth under your breast, or to use a scarf tied behind your neck as a sort of breast sling. Take care, though, that nothing is squashing or digging into your breast while your baby is feeding.

How to manage your clothes so your baby can feed

However you feed your baby, it's important that your clothes don't get in his way (or yours), or stop your breasts hanging freely. Your bra, if you wear one, should allow you to uncover each breast fully while feeding, so that its shape isn't distorted. If you choose to wear a normal bra instead of a nursing bra, undo it – or slip the strap off your shoulder – for feeding. Just lifting the cup from underneath is not a good idea because the tightness of the bra across the top of your breast could prevent it from draining properly, which in turn could lead to a blocked duct or mastitis. The same thing applies to a bikini top.

Is my baby feeding effectively?

The difference between a baby feeding effectively at the breast and one who is struggling to get milk is obvious – *if* you know what to look for. However, many people (parents, grandparents and health professionals) don't realise that breastfeeding is different from bottle feeding. So, when they see a baby 'sucking strongly' (usually with his lips pursed and cheeks drawn in), they assume he is feeding effectively. They couldn't be more wrong.

Here's what a baby who is feeding effectively at the breast looks like:

- His chin is pressed into the breast (because his head is tilted back).
- He has a wide-open mouth and (although you may not be able to see it) his bottom lip is curled back (because he attached with his chin leading).
- His cheeks are full and rounded (because his mouth is full of breast).
- More of his mother's areola is showing above his top lip than below his bottom lip (because her nipple is angled up towards his soft palate, right at the back of his mouth). (NB: If your areola is very small you probably won't be able to see any of it.)
- He sucks and swallows in a rhythmic way (see page 92).
- He lets go of the breast spontaneously when he's had enough (see page 94).

You can see most of these signs in photo number 18. Check for them yourself while your baby is feeding. (If you have large breasts and can't easily see your baby's mouth you may want to use a mirror, or get your partner or a friend to have a look.) If any sign is missing, it's likely that feeding is *not* effective, even if the other signs are present.

Two other signs of effective feeding are important:

- Your nipple should be the same shape and colour at the end of the feed as it was at the beginning (not squashed or pinched).
- Apart from a possible 'ouch!' moment at the beginning of the feed while you are both learning (see box on page 38), feeding should be pain free.

However, on their own pain-free feeding and undamaged nipples don't necessarily mean that all is well. Look for all the signs listed above, just to be sure.

Shutting your eyes occasionally while your baby is feeding will help you to learn what effective feeding feels and sounds like, so you don't always need to check what it looks like.

Take your time – and trust your baby

Breastfeeding takes time to learn. Even if you've done it before, it will be different with this new baby. And he needs to practise, too. Babies often wriggle around, attach, and let go a few times at the beginning of a feed, but eventually they find what feels right and settle down to a pattern of rhythmic sucking and swallowing. This fiddly bit will get shorter at each feed as your baby learns what to do, but in the meantime you'll need to be patient and let him work things out. If you try to help him by putting the breast in his mouth or holding his head, he's likely to become *more* frustrated, not less, because his instincts are telling him this isn't what's supposed to happen. If you've followed the *Essentials for helping your baby to feed* on page 43, your baby will do the rest.

Key points

- Ineffective attachment of the baby at the breast is the cause of most common breastfeeding problems.

- Babies have strong instincts to help them to breastfeed; your role is to make it easy for your baby to do what he needs to do, not to try to help him by doing it for him.

- Using bottles and dummies can interfere with babies' learning.

- Breastfeeding is different from bottle feeding and babies need to be held differently for each.

- A lying-back position can be helpful for learning.

- When holding your baby for feeding, focus on his needs first, then make yourself comfortable once he's feeding.

- Breastfeeding shouldn't hurt. Except for a few seconds at the very beginning of a feed in the early days, pain while feeding is a sign that something is wrong.

- You and baby need time to learn – together.

part II

What happens with baby-led breastfeeding

4

When your baby is born

Baby-led breastfeeding begins at birth. When a baby is born, both mother and baby are already primed with instincts and reflexes, ready for breastfeeding. These natural responses are triggered by skin-to-skin contact between them, and if this is not interrupted, breastfeeding happens naturally. Many mothers who didn't plan to breastfeed have been surprised at how right it can feel to let their newborn baby follow her instincts and feed.

Normal, healthy, full-term babies know how to breastfeed. Their drive to find the breast is at its strongest immediately after birth and gradually weakens in the hours and weeks that follow. This chapter is about how to support your baby to use her instincts and how to make the most of your first precious hours with her – as well as what to do if this can't happen.

Why skin-to-skin contact is so important

Skin-to-skin contact is the best way for breastfeeding to start. It's also enormously important for bonding with your baby, to help you both to feel safe and recover from the birth. When your naked baby is against your chest, surges of hormones are created, which tell your breasts to start making milk (see page 22). They also start the process of you falling in love with your baby and wanting to protect her.

For your baby, skin-to-skin contact is the nearest thing to when she was in the womb, so it helps her adjust to being outside your body. Being held skin to skin regulates her temperature; your chest is the warmest part of your body, so it's the best place for her to be to stop her getting cold. Skin-to-skin contact also allows your baby to pick up some of your natural skin bacteria, helping to protect her from infections. She will be able to hear your heartbeat and she'll recognise your voice. Your reassuring presence will help to steady her breathing and calm her. Just as you did before she was born, as a new mother you can provide everything she needs at this special time.

Skin-to-skin contact triggers the instincts that help babies to breastfeed:

- *Crawling to the breast:* Drawn by the unique scent produced by the glands around your nipples (which is similar to the smell of your amniotic fluid), your baby will instinctively press her feet and knees into you and push herself towards your breast. This instinct fades gradually in the first few weeks – by the time she is six weeks old she will have 'forgotten' how to crawl.

- *Finding the nipple:* When your baby's head brushes up against your breast she'll spontaneously lift or turn it to find your nipple. Then she'll tilt it back, open her mouth wide, and use her tongue to scoop up a big mouthful of breast. She may wriggle around and bob her head up and down several times before she gets it just right.

- *Starting to suck:* Once she's scooped up a mouthful of breast, your baby will automatically start to suck. And, because she has an innate preference for sweet tastes, she'll love the taste of your milk.

These instincts are strongest in the first hour or two after birth, so if both mother and baby are well this is the ideal time for them to be in skin-to-skin contact.

Your baby's first breastfeed

As soon as your baby is born – even before the placenta is delivered – ask your birth partner and your midwife to help you get comfortable lying back (supported by cushions or a bean bag) with your baby on top of you. You'll need to have your tummy and chest bare (no bra or top), though you may want something around your shoulders if the room is cool.

Your baby should be dried quickly – but not wrapped. With a blanket or towel over her back, she will be safe and warm. Make sure the cover isn't tight or too heavy, so that she can move her head and limbs easily. If the room is cool and her hair is damp, ask for a hat for her so that she doesn't lose heat. Photos number 1 to 4 and 12 shows a mother and baby skin to skin, just after the birth.

Let your baby take her time to discover the feel of your skin and your unique smell, and to crawl gradually towards your breast. Expect her to have short bursts of activity with periods of rest in between.

It usually takes at least half an hour – and often an hour or more – for a newborn baby to find her mother's breast and start to feed. There's no rush, though. Babies aren't born hungry; they have been fed through the umbilical cord right up until the point of birth. This first feed is a way for your baby to discover for herself what she needs to do, so that she knows how to latch on later, when she *is* hungry.

'Jake fed even before the placenta was delivered. The midwife lifted him on to my belly and within minutes he was obviously looking for something. He knew exactly where to go and what he wanted. He started feeding straight away – he just knew what to do. With Beth it was different. I didn't have skin to skin with her. When I offered her the breast she licked it and sniffed it, and nuzzled a bit, but she didn't feed properly for about 12 hours.'

Ruth, mother of Jake, two years, and Beth, six weeks

It's important that, as far as possible, no one and nothing interferes with your baby's instinctive behaviour. She is the one doing the feeding. You may need to support her weight a little but don't be tempted to help her to find your breast or open her mouth. Her head must be free to move and bob about – it shouldn't be held or pushed on to the breast – and she needs to be allowed to do things in her own time. If she is interrupted before she gets as far as feeding she will have to start again, right back at the beginning, slowing everything down and delaying her learning.

Letting your baby lead the way from the moment she's born will cement her instincts and make breastfeeding easier for both of you. Rushing her or trying to do it for her can make everything harder.

Giving your baby's instincts a chance

All new mothers and babies respond in similar ways when they are in skin-to-skin contact, because their hormones and instincts take over. It's important for those around them to help protect this special time and to prevent any interruptions. Others may be rushing about (especially in a busy maternity unit) but these precious moments only happen once for each mother and baby.

Old-fashioned midwifery care involved getting the baby into a cot as soon as possible so that the mother could rest, but as long as you are comfortable and there is someone with you to make sure your baby is safe if you drift off to sleep, having her with you, feeding, nuzzling or sleeping, will probably help you to relax more than being separated from her. This is partly because you'll know she's safe and partly because the hormones triggered by her closeness will help you feel relaxed and sleepy.

Skin contact shouldn't normally need to be postponed or interrupted in order for your baby to have a routine examination, while the placenta is delivered or while you have stitches put in. A skilled midwife can examine a baby while she is lying on her mother – and, provided your vaginal area is properly numbed, having your baby to cuddle can be a good way to take your mind off being stitched. **It's reasonable for you (or your birth partner) to challenge anyone who suggests interrupting your skin-to-skin contact with your baby unnecessarily.**

Aim to stay in skin-to-skin contact with your baby at least until she has had her first feed. If you have to be transferred to a different ward or room before that, ask if you can stay in skin contact during the move. If this isn't possible, start skin contact again as soon as you can – preferably before you have a bath or shower, so that you don't confuse her by changing how you smell.

It's helpful if your partner and other relatives understand in advance why it's so important that only *you* should be holding your baby for the first hours. Everyone wants to cuddle a new baby as soon as they can, but passing your baby round from one person to another while you and she are still getting to know each other will confuse her and may hamper breastfeeding. Let them know this time is the best time to get breastfeeding going well and for you and your baby to bond.

What about weighing my baby?

Most new parents are keen to know what their baby weighs but it can mean interrupting your time in skin contact. If weighing can't be postponed, perhaps because the midwife needs to complete the birth records promptly, the best alternative is to ask to have your baby weighed *as soon as she's born*. It will only take a few seconds to lift her into the scales and then back on to you – and it will mean she can then take all the time she needs to find your breast and have her first feed.

Can my partner have skin contact?

Skin-to-skin contact is a lovely way for a baby to bond with both her parents but there are two key reasons why you, as her mother, should be given priority to start with. Firstly, skin contact really is the best way to get going with breastfeeding and it can help you to avoid a lot of common problems later. Your baby's feeding instincts will never again be as strong as they are immediately after the birth, so it makes sense to make the most of them.

The second reason why the first skin-to-skin experience your baby has should be with you is that labour and birth are very stressful – and skin contact is the perfect way for both of you to relax, rest and recover. From your baby's point of view, she's been inside you all this time, so it's *you* she's expecting to meet; she wants to hear your voice and smell your scent – and it's *your* reward for all that hard work.

All of this doesn't mean your partner or birth companion has to be excluded – he or she can cuddle *both* of you. But at this special time, their main role is to keep you and your baby together and safe, and to speak up for you both if anyone tries to separate you. This is enormously important because it allows you to focus on your baby and tune in to her needs.

What if my baby is sleepy?

If you have been given pain-relieving injections or an epidural anaesthetic during labour your baby may well be born with some of the drugs still in her system. Her body will deal with this more slowly than yours, and she will probably be quite sleepy – perhaps for a couple of days.

If your baby is drowsy when she's born it's especially important that her skin-to-skin contact with you is not interrupted until she's had her first feed. Babies who are sleepy at birth usually take longer to find the breast and start feeding – as much as two or three hours. It may seem as though she is not interested and it can be tempting to put her in a cot to sleep it off. But babies who are sedated by drugs can sleep for hours, and if they are not in contact with their mother their instinct to search for the breast can start to weaken. It's not unusual to have problems getting breastfeeding going when this has been allowed to happen.

What if things are complicated?

Not all births are straightforward, so skin contact and early feeds sometimes have to be adapted. If the baby has been born very early (or if either mother or baby is ill) skin-to-skin time may even have to be put on hold (see Chapter 11). But if both are well it should still be possible, even if there have been complications around the time of the birth.

The first feed for twins or triplets

How ready newborn twins or triplets are to breastfeed depends on how mature they are. Multiples are often born early, and premature babies may need special care following the birth (see Chapter 11). But if they are well enough to be with you, having skin contact with more than one baby shouldn't be a problem, with a little help.

If your babies are born normally you may have the opportunity for a quick cuddle with the one who arrives first.

However, you will need to hand him or her to your birth partner when the second one is ready to be born so that you can concentrate on pushing. Once the birth is over, you'll probably need a little help to position your babies on your tummy and stop them from falling but that's really the only challenge – they are used to sharing a cramped space.

Like any other babies, full-term multiples can feed themselves, if given the opportunity. They may be ready to feed at the same time but there's every chance that one will lead the way. Either way, if the babies are well there's no need to rush to get it all to happen quickly.

'After the twins were born I let each baby crawl up to the breast in turn. It was very slow because they were so sleepy but they found their way, latched on and had a feed. When the first was finished I gave her to my husband and did the same with the other one. They were just like little newborn animals – it was wonderful.'

Sam, mother of George, four years, Zoe and Ellen, two years

If it's a difficult birth

Unless you are ill, or your baby needs special care (see page 185), skin-to-skin contact is the best way for both of you to recover from a difficult birth. However, it's especially important to have someone else there to make sure you are both safe if you are very tired, weak from losing blood, or if an anaesthetic has left you woozy or unable to move much.

Your baby may have bruising and a headache, especially if she was born with the help of a vacuum pump or forceps. This is likely to make her irritable, especially if her head is handled in an effort to help her to feed. Letting her take her time to feed, preferably on top of you, with you in a lying-back position, will mean her head is less likely to be touched.

If being born has been a struggle it's quite likely your baby will be too exhausted to feed at first. If your midwife or

IF YOU ARE OVERWEIGHT

If you are very overweight you may be more likely to have a complicated birth and experience a delayed start to milk production. Spending lots of time in skin-to-skin contact with your baby and asking for help to find feeding positions that work for you both will give you the best chance of getting breastfeeding going well.

paediatrician feels she needs food quickly, you can express some of your milk for her. Because the first milk, colostrum, is thick, it's easy to do this by hand (see page 86), even if you're lying down. Ask for help if you need it. You can express the milk either directly on to your baby's lips, on to your fingertip, or, if she needs medical attention, into a small syringe, so she can have it straight away.

After a Caesarean section

Having a Caesarean section doesn't necessarily mean you and your baby can't have skin contact immediately; it all depends on whether or not you are awake during the birth and how well you both are. Nowadays many hospitals are keen for mothers who have a Caesarean section under an epidural anaesthetic to hold their baby while the surgery is being finished, and it's usually possible for this to be skin to skin.

Operating tables aren't very roomy, so the time you spend in the recovery room may be a better opportunity for quality skin-to-skin contact. It's likely to last longer then, too, so your baby can have her first breastfeed undisturbed. Your birth partner can play a big part in helping you to lie comfortably and hold your baby safely, especially if you are coming round from a general anaesthetic.

Some mothers who have a Caesarean section find that their milk production takes a while to get going. Spending plenty of time in skin-to-skin contact with your baby after this type of birth can make a huge difference to your chances of a successful start with breastfeeding.

'Lola was born by C-section and she had skin to skin straight away – she was just laid on top of me and she fed for a good half an hour while I was being stitched. I was the last op of the day and no emergencies came in so we had plenty of time. Now I usually feed Lola like that first thing in the morning. I lie back on the pillows and she just finds the nipple herself and gets on with it.'

Rebecca, *mother of Lola, 11 weeks*

If you or your baby are unwell

Sometimes it isn't possible for mother and baby to have skin contact immediately after the birth: for example, if the baby is born very prematurely (see Chapter 11) and needs to go straight into an incubator, or if she needs to be given oxygen. Such circumstances may mean that skin contact has to be delayed – but it doesn't mean it can't happen at all. And it certainly doesn't mean that breastfeeding won't be possible.

If skin contact has to be postponed because *you* are unwell, your baby can have it with your birth partner instead. This will calm and comfort her and enable the two of them to begin their own bonding. Meanwhile, expressing some colostrum will help to kick-start your milk production as well as providing food for your baby (see page 187).

If you can't spend time skin to skin with your baby as soon as she's born, be sure to let the hospital staff know that you want to do this as soon as possible and try to make sure that your first breastfeed together – however much later this is – starts this way. You may also want to discuss ways of feeding your baby in the meantime that will interfere as little as possible with her instincts to breastfeed (see *Feeding your baby before he is ready to breastfeed*, page 192).

The first 48 hours

The first day or two after your baby's birth can be a bit daunting, especially if you are in hospital. Some hospitals and birthing centres allow partners to stay round the clock but it's more common for them to be asked to leave, especially at night. So it's a good idea to think ahead about what will make it easier for you to respond to your baby, if there's no one right by you to help.

> 'It was hard the first night in hospital. I lay staring at Maya in her little cot and I kept putting my hand on her to check she was breathing. I was so worried each time she woke up because it meant I had to get her out of the cot and try to feed her. I just didn't have a clue what to do.'
>
> *Safiya, mother of Maya, three months*

You are likely to be exhausted in the first few hours after giving birth and you may have drugs in your system that make it unsafe for your baby to stay in your bed. However, you won't want to move far to reach her – especially if you are finding moving difficult. You'll also want to be sure of waking quickly when she needs you. Many hospitals have cots that clip on to the mother's bed but if that option isn't available (and it's worth asking, just in case) ask your birth partner to help you get your baby's cot as close to your bed as possible, so that you can reach her easily and lift her out for feeding (and put her back) with the least effort.

Laying your baby skin to skin on your tummy for feeds will make feeding more instinctive for both of you. It will also avoid you having to work out how to hold her and how to get the timing right for latching on because she'll do most of it by herself. However, if you are sore or have stitches, you may find it difficult to get comfortable. If you're prepared to be inventive, and can get someone to help you lift her and move pillows or cushions to where you need them, you'll be able to find a position for feeding that works. It doesn't matter if it's unconventional – what's important is how your baby is positioned against your body (see page 42), not whether you are sitting or lying in a certain way. Don't be afraid to ask for painkillers to help you move more easily.

Some women feel slightly jittery in the day or two following their baby's birth, and find it difficult to sleep; others feel overwhelmingly tired and are nervous about sleeping too deeply. Don't be afraid to ask a member of staff to wake you if necessary to feed your baby, and to come and check on you both later, in case you fall asleep during the feed.

Unless you or your baby is ill, there should be no need for anyone to suggest taking her away from you at any time, including during the night.

If your baby needs encouragement to feed

Not all babies feed frequently on the first day and some have as few as three feeds in the first 24 hours. Provided your baby has had a feed within an hour or two after birth, this won't usually be considered a problem. But from the second day onwards she should be showing signs of wanting to feed more frequently. If this isn't happening by the time she's a day and a half old (perhaps because she is very sleepy, either recovering from the birth or sleeping off the effects of drugs you were given in labour) it's probably a good idea to start offering her the breast more often – even if she seems to be asleep.

Babies' instincts are so strong that the smell and feel of their mother's breast tends to make them want to breastfeed even if they haven't got the energy to do anything else. Holding your baby skin to skin, and expressing a little milk on to her lips may be enough to tempt her to latch on. If not, ask your midwife for help to give her some expressed milk in a cup or syringe.

If you have diabetes

If you have diabetes your baby is likely to need some extra feeds, while her metabolism is adjusting to being outside the womb. To avoid her being given formula (which may – according to some research – trigger diabetes later in childhood) you will probably be encouraged to express and save your colostrum for her towards the end of pregnancy.

Making sure you have a snack whenever she feeds will help to prevent you having a hypoglycaemic 'dip' afterwards.

Key points

- Uninterrupted skin-to-skin contact as soon as possible after the birth is the best way for breastfeeding to start.

- A lying-back position, with your baby on top of you, will allow her to use her instincts for her very first feed.

- Your baby knows what to do. Let her lead the way and try not to interrupt her or interfere.

- Relax – it can take an hour or more for a newborn baby to find the breast and start to feed.

- Don't wash your breasts until your baby has fed at least once, so she can recognise your smell.

- Your birth partner can make sure skin-to-skin contact is not interrupted until your baby has had her first feed (and for as long as possible after that).

- If skin-to-skin contact can't happen immediately after the birth it can still happen later.

- Don't be afraid to ask for the help you need in the first few days to care for your baby and hold her for feeding.

5

The first two weeks

The first two weeks after a baby's birth are a period of huge physical and emotional adjustment, even for experienced parents. Adapting to a new baby in the family, getting to grips with his needs and recovering from the birth all present their own challenges.

These two weeks are also crucial for breastfeeding. Frequent and effective feeding during this time lays the foundations for long-term stress-free feeding and optimum milk production. In many cases where breastfeeding goes wrong, the problem can be traced back to this very early period.

Investing plenty of time at this stage, so you can learn how to interpret your baby's signals and follow his lead, will help you to avoid the sort of difficulties that so many mothers and babies encounter. This chapter explains how.

Having a babymoon

The first two weeks of breastfeeding can be thought of like a honeymoon, only with your baby as the focus of your attention. The idea is to concentrate on getting to know him, and on breastfeeding, with as few distractions and other responsibilities as possible. Some people call this a 'babymoon'.

The essence of a babymoon is spending as much time as you can holding your baby skin to skin. Keeping him against the warmth of your chest, where he can nuzzle your breast and feed whenever he wants, will make the most of his instincts. It will also cause surges of prolactin and oxytocin, triggering milk production and your instinct to nurture him, and making the adjustment to motherhood easier.

A babymoon relies on your partner, family or friends helping with meals and housework, so you can focus mainly on your baby. It doesn't necessarily mean you have to be secluded or stay indoors as long as you can spend time getting to know your baby. It works best if you establish a kind of 'nest' for you and your baby – maybe in bed or on the sofa – that's comfortable and easy for feeding (but see page 115 for important safety information). If you have an older child or children, spending time with them will be important (especially if they are still breastfeeding) but your newborn needs to be your priority.

Getting to know your baby can be easier if you don't have lots of people dropping in to visit – especially if you are likely to feel inhibited about breastfeeding in front of them. Limiting visitors for a week or two (or limiting how long they stay) will also prevent your baby being passed around and fussed over, which may tire him out or lead to his feeding cues going unnoticed – especially if whoever is holding him thinks babies don't need to be fed unless they cry. Many new mothers find that a day with lots of visitors leaves them exhausted, with painfully full breasts and a fractious baby who has difficulty latching on. Try to stay near your baby whenever anyone else is holding him, so that you can spot when he needs you and feed him promptly.

A babymoon allows you to get confident with breastfeeding in your own time, without having to worry about who's watching and whether you're doing it 'right'. This will make it much easier, later on, to feed your baby when there are other people around and to resist well-meant but unhelpful advice.

'I had all my visitors on the day I came home and Ben just slept through it, in my arms. After that we didn't see anyone for about

10 days. I stayed in my pyjamas and the three of us spent a lot of time in bed, with Ben feeding and us gazing at him. It felt like it was our time to knit together as a family – I wouldn't give it back for anything. And by the time people started saying things like "Are you sure he's getting enough?" I was confident enough not to take any notice.'

Caroline, mother of Ben, five years

It's a good idea to warn your friends and relatives in advance if you plan to limit visitors at first, and explain to them why this is important to you. There will be plenty of opportunities later for them to get to know your baby but these first two weeks are your best chance to get breastfeeding going well.

Putting in the order for milk

The first two weeks of breastfeeding establish your potential for long-term milk production. The more your baby breast-feeds during this time the more milk you will make now – and the more you will be able to make later, whenever it's needed. **Your breastmilk is all he needs unless there is a genuine medical reason for him to be given something else.** Formula or water will fill up his tummy and dampen his keenness to breastfeed.

Bottles and dummies are best avoided, too. A dummy may make your baby sleep longer than he should or prevent you from spotting that he needs to feed, meaning that breastfeeds are delayed or missed, while giving him anything in a bottle – even your expressed breastmilk – may interfere with the way he uses his mouth to breastfeed.

The acronym **FEEDS** is an easy way to remember what's important, especially in the early weeks. To give you and your baby the best start, breastfeeding needs to be:

- **F**requent: day and night – expect your baby to feed *at least* eight times every 24 hours in the first two weeks (and probably more, especially if some feeds are very short) and *at least* six times every 24 hours after that.

- **E**ffective: with your baby attached so that he can get milk easily.

- **E**xclusive: with your baby having only your milk – no other drinks or food, not even water.

- *On* **D**emand: whenever your baby asks – or sooner, if he's sleepy or your breasts are uncomfortably full – and for as long as he wants each time.

- **S**kin to skin as much as possible, in the early weeks.

'Jude was always a hungry baby and fed a lot. I loved that lazy and relaxed pace of life. I'd spend all afternoon on the sofa feeding – it was all about nurturing him. He was born on the 91st centile and never lost any weight. He was just getting what he needed.'

Anka, mother of Jude, two years

Frequent breastfeeding is good for you and your baby

Lots of small feeds allow your baby to learn to co-ordinate his breathing with sucking and swallowing. They also allow his stomach (which is about the size of a marble at birth) to stretch gently. Colostrum, with its highly concentrated nourishment, is the perfect food for the first few days and, if he feeds frequently, your baby will be able to adjust as the volume of milk increases – and he'll stop you getting overfull.

Frequent breastfeeding in the beginning also makes a difference to how well your baby adapts to life outside the womb. Research shows that, compared with babies who have few feeds, those who breastfeed frequently from birth:

- lose less weight in their first week
- have less jaundice (see page 84), and
- stimulate their mothers to make more milk.

Frequent breastfeeding will also:

- prevent you from becoming engorged (see page 235), keeping you comfortable and making it easier for your baby to latch on
- establish your long-term ability to make plenty of milk
- give you and your baby lots of opportunities to practise breastfeeding instinctively, with less time between feeds to forget what you need to do.

The frequency of your baby's feeds is likely to reach a peak around the fifth day, when it may feel as though he is *always* wanting milk. After that, things will gradually settle into a pattern, though this will be different for every baby. Some feeds will be long, others just snacks – but you can expect your baby to feed *at least* eight times a day in the early weeks, and quite possibly 12 or more.

ADULTS FEED FREQUENTLY TOO!

A breastfeed is food *and* drink for babies. If you add up all your own snacks, meals and drinks you may be surprised how often you have a 'feed'. You probably don't eat at regular intervals, or go for very long without a little something, and the amount you consume – and how quickly you do it – will vary each time. You may even find that, except at night, you feed *more* often than your newborn.

'Sometimes Chana used to feed for a while then fall asleep and want to feed again 15 or 20 minutes later. She seemed quite happy with it but I was stressed thinking she needed another feed so quickly. I didn't realise it was probably the same feed. She was having a little break – just as we would in a restaurant before the dessert.'

Jazmin, mother of Chana, 16 months

Feeding isn't just about hunger

Your baby doesn't have to be hungry or thirsty to want – and need – a breastfeed. Breastfeeding provides babies with comfort, warmth and security as well as food and drink – and it's impossible to over-feed a breastfed baby. If your baby is asking to feed and you think he can't possibly be hungry again, you may be right – but that doesn't mean he doesn't need to feed. Responding to your baby's requests will make both parenting and breastfeeding easier.

Babies need to feed through the night as well as during the day, and night feeds can be as unpredictable as daytime feeds, at least in the first few weeks. Many exhausted new parents find this one of the hardest things to adjust to, but the more practice with feeding you and your baby have during the day, the easier night feeds will become. Once you don't need to concentrate so much to breastfeed you won't need to wake up properly or put the light on to do it at night. (See page 113 for more on night feeds.)

Understanding your baby

Part of getting to know your baby is understanding how he communicates and what he is trying to tell you. In the first couple of weeks, most of his requests will relate to his needs for feeding and security, because survival is his priority. Keeping your baby next to you, night and day, will enable you to spot when he wants to feed and make caring for him much easier.

Feeding your baby when he is only just stirring means he is likely to attach to the breast more easily. You'll soon find that your let-down reflex happens before you've even picked him up, which means that he doesn't have to wait for food to be available and learns to trust you to be there when he needs you.

Knowing when your baby needs to feed

Babies let their parents know that they want to feed through a variety of 'feeding cues' but some are very subtle and it's easy to miss them. If a baby is asking for a feed and no one responds, eventually he will cry. **Many people think crying is the only way babies tell us they want to feed but in fact it is a baby's final attempt to get his message across to someone who can help.** From the baby's point of view it's all about survival, so his desperation is genuine.

Waiting until a baby cries before feeding him makes breastfeeding unnecessarily difficult. Here's why:

- Crying gets in the way of latching on, so it can prevent the baby from feeding effectively.
- Crying gives babies wind, which can make them uncomfortable after a feed.
- Crying makes babies stressed, causing them to get frustrated at the breast and making it difficult for them to feed in a relaxed way.

It's not just the baby who gets stressed if his cues are ignored. Listening to a baby cry, even for a few minutes, is stressful for the adults around him. It's *supposed* to be like this because it's an alarm to warn the mother her baby needs her. Answering your baby before he gets upset will help him to feel safe, as well as making feeding easier.

Recognising when your baby needs to feed involves watching and listening to him carefully, especially while you're still getting to know each other. His first signals are likely to be very fleeting (see box, below). If he is not offered a feed fairly quickly he will become more active until eventually, if he's still ignored, he will move on to crying.

Some babies are very sleepy for several days after birth (see page 60) and don't get past the murmuring stage before going back into a deep sleep. It's especially important for someone to recognise these very subtle cues, so the baby doesn't miss out on the chance to feed.

Dummies (or pacifiers) can prevent some feeding cues, such as sucking movements, from being spotted. And some babies will find a dummy so soothing that they drift back off to sleep without anyone knowing that they needed to feed. Long gaps between feeds send messages to the breasts to slow down milk production, which can mean the baby doesn't get enough milk to put on weight.

Keeping your baby close will allow you to spot his earliest feeding cues. The sooner you notice that he wants to feed, the more chance you'll have to finish what you're doing or get

---

Early cues that your baby wants to feed

- Moving his eyes under his eyelids.
- Moving his head and stretching his neck.
- Making gentle wriggling, squirming and waving movements.
- Clenching and unclenching his fists.
- Opening his mouth and making 'rooting' movements (see *Your baby knows how to breastfeed*, page 35).
- Making sucking noises or smacking his lips.
- Murmuring, squeaking, whimpering or giving little shouts.
- Sucking his fists/clothes/blanket, or your T-shirt/jumper.

yourself a drink before he starts to get distressed, so that you can settle down for a relaxed feed. At night, these early signals will give you a chance to come round enough to feed him without either of you needing to wake up fully.

Babies don't have to be very hungry to want to breastfeed. After all, they aren't born hungry, but they still have a very strong instinct to go to the breast straight after birth (see page 56). Carrying your baby in your arms or in a sling, or having him lie beside you in bed at night (see page 114), will mean you feel his smallest movements and get the earliest possible signal that he would like to feed.

Letting your baby lead the way means not making him wait to feed – but it doesn't mean you always have to wait for him to ask. If you become engorged, you'll be in pain and he'll find it hard to attach. So, if your breasts feel uncomfortably full, it's in your baby's interests as well as yours to offer him the chance to feed a bit earlier than he'd planned.

'Emily wasn't happy for the first month or two. In retrospect it's obvious I just wasn't feeding her enough. I'd feed her and sometimes she'd want more 20 minutes later. I'd see all the signs but I didn't believe she needed it so I'd try to jiggle her to stop her crying. So she was miserable a lot of the time. I knew feeding her would work but it felt like cheating – it was too easy.'

Jane, mother of Emily, five years

What else your baby can tell you

Breastfeeding is a skill you and your baby have to learn together. Part of trusting him to lead the way is recognising his feeding cues and respecting his instinctive knowledge of what to do at the breast. But the other part is recognising when he's trying to tell you that something is wrong.

Some babies who are finding breastfeeding difficult try to signal to their mothers by squirming, pulling on and off the

ONE BREAST OR TWO?

Whether your baby feeds from one breast or both at each feed is up to him and how hungry or thirsty he is. Just let him feed for as long as he wants on the first breast and then, when he lets go, offer him the second. If he still seems hungry after that, try him on the first again.

It doesn't really matter which one he starts with each time, but feeding from the fuller one first will be best for your comfort. If your baby has a favourite breast it's likely to make more milk and may be noticeably bigger than the other one in the early weeks, especially just before a feed. The difference will soon become much less obvious and once breastfeeding is over, both breasts will return to the same size.

FEED BEFORE YOU GET FULL

It can be tempting to make your baby wait until your breasts feel really full before letting him feed but this won't encourage him to take more milk or sleep longer between feeds; it's more likely to make him fretful and lead to him having difficulty latching on or coping with the milk flow. *Not* waiting until your breasts are overfull – or your baby is desperately hungry – before you let him feed is one of the secrets of effortless and relaxed breastfeeding.

breast and crying (they are often labelled 'difficult feeders' or 'breast refusers'). Others just resign themselves to the situation, becoming lethargic and reluctant to feed. Often, the problem isn't spotted until someone notices that the baby isn't gaining weight. If your instinct tells you something isn't right, ask for help (see *Where can I get help?*, page 106).

Your breasts in the first two weeks

Your breasts probably won't feel very different for a day or so after your baby is born but there is a lot going on inside them: the blood supply is increasing and surges of prolactin are prompting the milk-making cells into full-scale production. After a day or two, you may notice the thick, concentrated colostrum gradually changing, becoming more watery and less yellow, and your breasts may start to feel full.

Breastmilk doesn't suddenly 'come in' on the third day, and your breasts shouldn't be hard, swollen, shiny or red, although they may be tender. 'Third-day engorgement' used to be thought of as normal just because most mothers experienced it. However, it was actually the result of restricting breastfeeds to every four hours and taking babies away from their mothers (and giving them formula) at night.

Allowing your breasts to become overfull will not only be painful for you but will also make it difficult for your baby to latch on, so if you do start to feel uncomfortable, just offer your baby a feed. If he seems to be struggling to attach, hand express a little milk (see page 86) to soften your breast and make it easier for him.

It can take a week or two for your let-down reflex (see page 24) to work in sync with your baby. Until then it's likely to be erratic. It's normal for it to happen at odd times for no particular reason, or to take a while to work when your baby is at your breast. Offering your baby the chance to feed whenever you notice a tingling sensation or a sudden leakage of milk will help it begin to work more reliably. Once your body has learnt what to do you may find that the reflex is triggered just by thinking about feeding your baby, or by hearing him (or someone else's baby) cry.

In the first two weeks, your breasts will normally feel fuller before a feed than they do afterwards but this will change as they start to respond more accurately to your baby's needs (see page 122). It's a good idea to get used to handling them so that you can detect any problems early (see *Painful breastfeeding: quick symptom checker*, page 275).

What can I do about leaking milk?

Some women never leak milk, others leak often and some leak more from one breast than the other. It's particularly common to leak milk when the let-down reflex operates, especially in the early weeks. (If your baby is feeding when this happens, you can expect the other breast to leak.)

If you know you're prone to leaking you'll probably want to wear breast pads (commercial or home-made), so that you don't get damp patches. Something thick and absorbent, which allows the skin to breathe, is better than something with a plastic backing, which may make a thrush infection (see page 232) more likely.

If you leak profusely from one breast while feeding from the other, you may find a drip catcher (a rigid plastic shell-shaped gadget that you put inside your bra) more effective than a breast pad. Be careful to check that the pouring spout is at the top! If you make sure the drip catcher is thoroughly

---

TIPS FOR MANAGING UNEXPECTED LEAKS

- If you feel your let-down reflex starting to work at an inconvenient moment, pressing the heels of your hands against your breasts may be enough to stop it in its tracks. If you're in company you can probably do this discreetly, just by folding your arms or pressing your elbow against your breast. (You can fiddle with an earring, so it's not obvious.)
- Wearing a loose, patterned top rather than a tight, plain one will mean the odd damp patch is less noticeable.

clean beforehand, you'll be able to save the milk you collect. It's not a good idea to wear a drip catcher *between* feeds, since they tend to press into the breasts and encourage even more leakage.

If your milk flows too rapidly for your baby

It's quite common for babies to struggle to cope with the flow of milk in the first few weeks, especially at the beginning of a feed when the let-down reflex is at its strongest. Sometimes one breast has faster flow than the other. If your baby pulls away from the breast coughing and spluttering there are several things you can do to help him:

- Take your baby off the breast for a few seconds when you feel the let-down reflex starting, then let him feed again once it's died down. If he seems uncomfortable, hold him upright for a few minutes so that he can bring up any air he may have swallowed.
- Express some milk before your baby begins feeding, to trigger the reflex. Wait until the flow subsides (or the tingling sensation stops) before offering him the breast.
- Hold your baby in a lying-back feeding position (as in photo number 21), so that his head is higher than your breast (sometimes referred to as feeding 'uphill'). This will lessen the force of the flow and make it easier for

SUCKING BLISTERS

Many babies develop sucking blisters – especially on their top lip – in the first week or so of breastfeeding, while they are getting the hang of it. The blisters don't seem to bother them and they don't need any treatment. They soon disappear.

him to clear his airway if he does start to splutter. Sitting him upright, straddling your thigh, to feed can help, too (see photo number 30).

Wind and bringing up milk

Babies burp, pass wind and bring up milk as a normal part of feeding, whether they are breastfed or formula fed. It can help to understand why this happens – and what, if anything, you need to do about it.

Do I need to wind my baby?

Breastfed babies don't usually need winding after feeds. They may swallow small amounts of air as they feed but this usually comes up by itself, as a burp. If your baby is settled and calm after a feed (and particularly if he has fallen asleep while feeding), there is no need to disturb him by rubbing or banging him vigorously on the back. If he *does* have any wind, it isn't causing him a problem and he will get rid of it on his own.

Babies are more likely to swallow air while they're feeding if their attachment at the breast is ineffective or if the flow of milk is very fast. They also swallow air as they cry. If your baby is struggling to cope with a rush of milk or has had to wait for his feed he may need the chance to bring up wind after the first few minutes. (See above for tips on dealing with a rapid milk flow.) Just sitting him upright or holding him against your shoulder will usually be enough to help him burp. Over-vigorous winding can make problems such as possetting and reflux (see below) worse.

Like adults, babies also make gas in their gut while they're digesting their food (including breastmilk). Gas can't be brought upwards by 'winding' – it has to go downwards.

Babies don't usually pass much more gas than their parents and it rarely causes them pain.

Is it normal for babies to be sick?

Most babies bring up small amounts of milk from their stomachs when they burp. Technically, this is called gastro-oesophageal reflux (GOR or GER), but it's more commonly known as possetting or spitting up. It's the same thing as when your own food repeats on you. Because a baby's oesophagus (the tube that goes from the mouth to the stomach) is much shorter than an adult's, some of the milk comes out of the top rather than going back down again.

Possetting can be a bit messy and inconvenient but it rarely worries babies (and regurgitated breastmilk doesn't smell sour). It is usually a sign that they have had a particularly large feed, or possibly that they've fed very fast. It's also more common when the baby has to gulp the milk, for example, if the flow is very fast (see page 80).

WHAT IS REFLUX DISEASE?

Some babies regurgitate their stomach contents so often that the lining of their oesophagus is damaged. This condition is called gastro-oesophageal reflux disease (GORD or GERD). It can lead to pain (and crying) during and after feeds, as well as breathing difficulties, poor weight gain and breast refusal. Some babies that are labelled as having colic in fact have GORD (GERD).

Thickeners (given before a breastfeed) are sometimes recommended for babies with GORD (GERD). However, while these reduce the amount of milk the baby brings right up, they don't actually stop the regurgitation, so they don't prevent damage to the oesophagus. There is a specific medicine that can help, but eventually babies outgrow the condition.

PROJECTILE VOMITING

Projectile vomiting can be a sign of pyloric stenosis, in which the muscle at the lower end of the stomach is unusually tight. If the stomach gets overfull, the contents get thrown back up forcefully. (Forceful vomiting can sometimes accompany a stomach infection but in that case the baby will have other signs of illness.) If vomiting is severe and frequent, the baby may not be able to keep enough milk down to gain weight. Sometimes the condition can be treated with medication to relax the muscle but it may require a small operation.

Just occasionally, what appears to be simply possetting is actually something more serious, such as reflux disease or the projectile vomiting of pyloric stenosis (see boxes above). Both of these are more likely to be a problem if the baby is formula fed than if he is breastfed, partly because formula is digested less quickly than breastmilk, and partly because formula feeds tend to be bigger and farther apart, causing the stomach to become over-stretched. Small, frequent feeds of breastmilk are generally easier for all babies to manage.

Pressure on the stomach, such as when a baby is sitting slumped in a car seat, makes possetting more likely and can make the symptoms of reflux worse. For the first half an hour after feeding, your baby may be more comfortable in an upright position, with his legs dangling, than either propped up or lying down, and so a sling may be useful.

If you have any concerns about the amount of milk your baby is bringing up, discuss it with your health visitor or doctor.

Newborn jaundice – what's normal and what isn't

It's common for babies to develop mild jaundice on their second or third day because their livers aren't very efficient at filtering a substance called bilirubin (produced by the breakdown of excess red blood cells) from their blood. Jaundice causes the skin and the whites of the eyes to get a yellowy tinge but it is not usually serious.

If the baby is feeding well he will be pooing frequently, which gets rid of bilirubin, so the jaundice will disappear quickly (usually by the end of the first week). However, if he isn't taking much milk, some of the bilirubin will be reabsorbed from his gut and the jaundice will take longer to clear. Unfortunately, jaundiced babies tend to be sleepy, so they don't ask for feeds as often as they should (and they may not feed effectively). This can lead to a vicious cycle, in which the mother's breasts aren't given enough stimulation and milk production goes down – which means the baby gets even less milk and the jaundice gets worse.

If breastfeeding gets off to a good start, jaundice is unlikely to be a problem and feeding can be baby-led. But if your baby is jaundiced and not feeding frequently – especially if he isn't producing many wees and poos (see page 97) – you will need to encourage him to feed more often (see *If your baby needs encouragement to feed*, page 66). When he does attach, check that he is feeding effectively (see page 49 – ask someone who knows about breastfeeding if you're unsure). Persuading him to take even small amounts of milk will give him more energy for feeding *and* help to get rid of the jaundice; simply waiting for his appetite to improve won't do either.

Depending on the severity of the jaundice, your midwife may refer your baby to a doctor, who may suggest ultraviolet light therapy (phototherapy) to help reduce the jaundice. Being under a warm light for long periods of time can make a baby dehydrated, so frequent breastfeeding is even more important.

Formula is sometimes suggested for jaundiced babies, to 'flush their system through' and get rid of the bilirubin. This is unnecessary. Colostrum has a laxative effect so it is just as good as formula at encouraging babies to poo frequently.

> 'Ella got jaundice and was put in an incubator. I was told to give her some formula because she needed lots of liquid. I gave her two formula feeds but I was so upset. After that I breastfed her every hour. I'd get her out of the incubator and hold her skin to skin with a blanket round us both and she'd feed. I think being a second-time mum I had the confidence to follow my instincts. She didn't need formula – she was fine and she's fed really well since then.'
>
> *Sharon, mother of Daniel, five years, and Ella, seven weeks*

So-called 'breastmilk jaundice' is much less common than newborn jaundice. It occurs only in breastfeeding babies and it doesn't usually appear until the baby is about two weeks old. The cause isn't fully understood but some mothers find it happens in all their babies.

Unlike a baby with prolonged newborn jaundice, the baby with breastmilk jaundice is alert, asking for feeds frequently, weeing and pooing normally and gaining weight. So, although it can last for several weeks or even months, this type of jaundice doesn't usually need any treatment. However, it can overlap with newborn jaundice if the newborn type is slow to clear because of ineffective or infrequent feeding. If your baby hasn't had a period *without* jaundice, the first thing to check is that he's getting enough milk.

Occasionally, a baby will develop jaundice for another reason, such as an infection or a problem with his liver. If your midwife or doctor suspects that your baby's jaundice may be anything other than normal, they will organise tests to find out what's wrong.

Learning to hand express your breastmilk

Expressing milk by hand is easy to do and can be useful in lots of ways. For example, in the early days it can help to relieve an overfull breast so that your baby can feed easily; later on it can be used to clear a blocked duct (see page 238).

Hand expression tends to be better than a breast pump at triggering the release of hormones (helping milk production and flow) and it can be gentler, too. Some women find it quicker, even for expressing large amounts (for example, for a premature baby, see page 187, or to leave with a babysitter, see Chapter 9), because there is no equipment to sterilise or assemble. You can do it whenever you need to and wherever you are; it costs nothing and you always have it – literally – at your fingertips.

The first two weeks are an ideal opportunity to practise hand expressing, so that you have the knack when you need to use it. Sometimes mothers are advised *not* to express in the first six weeks. However, it's not the expressing that's the problem – it's giving expressed milk *by bottle* while a baby is learning to breastfeed (see *Breastfeeding is different from bottle feeding*, page 34). You can express your milk as early as you like.

How to express your milk by hand

Before you start, you may need to stimulate your let-down reflex to get your milk flowing, by thinking about your baby or *gently* massaging or stroking your breast. There's no need to massage or stroke in a particular way, just do whatever feels nice. Don't expect much milk the first time you express – it can take some practice. (The tips on page 87 will help if you want to express lots of milk.)

When you express your milk by hand you are mimicking what your baby does with his mouth when he feeds (see page 32). Just like him, you need to find a spot a little way back from the nipple to squeeze the ducts so that the milk comes out. Here's how to do it:

1) Cup your breast in your (clean) hand with your thumb on top, in a C shape. (It's usually easiest to use the right hand on the right breast and the left hand on the left.)
2) Position your thumb and forefinger above and below your nipple, about 2cm (1 in) away from it.
3) Gently press your thumb and forefinger together. You should feel some breast tissue between them (it may feel gristly or lumpy). If all you feel is loose skin, try again, this time pressing backwards into your breast before you squeeze. Experiment with moving your finger and thumb slightly farther back from the nipple until you find the right spot. There is normally no need to go farther back than your baby reaches with his mouth when he feeds.
4) Now squeeze slightly more firmly, to compress the ducts. Release, then squeeze again (without dragging your fingers across your skin). Build up a rhythm of press and release.
5) If you are squeezing in the right place, you'll begin to see drops of milk emerging. If your baby is more than a few days old, you may even get fine jets or squirts (as in photo number 5). If you don't see anything after a few squeezes, experiment with moving your thumb and finger closer to the nipple or farther away.
6) Once you know how far from your nipple your fingers need to be, pressing in different places around an imaginary circle will get milk from all parts of the breast. If you have a blocked duct or mastitis, placing your thumb on the red or lumpy side of the breast will target that area (see also Chapter 13).

If all you want to do is soften an overfull breast so your baby can attach, a few squeezes at two or three different spots on your imaginary circle will probably be enough. If you want to express lots of milk, just keep going in one position until the flow subsides before moving to the next.

If you don't need to save the milk, you can express into any container or just over the sink. If you do want to keep the milk, use a thoroughly clean bowl or jug to catch it. (Breastmilk often squirts in different directions so choose a wide one.) If you are expressing for a preterm or ill baby, make sure the container you use is sterilised beforehand. See page 149 for information on storing breastmilk.

From now on it gets easier

The first two weeks of breastfeeding can be pretty full on and at times it will feel as though you're doing nothing but feeding. But once this time is over both you and your baby will be getting to grips with the practicalities of feeding and learning to trust each other. From now on his feeds will still need to be **F**requent, **E**ffective, **E**xclusive and on **D**emand (see page 71) – and **S**kin to skin, when you get the chance – but, as you and he get more in tune with each other and your confidence grows, you'll find yourself feeding him without even thinking about it.

It may not feel like a huge milestone but by focusing on breastfeeding for these two weeks you have set up your long-term capacity to produce as much milk as your baby needs and laid the foundations for an easy breastfeeding relationship.

Key points

- Having a two-week babymoon after your baby is born can make concentrating on breastfeeding easier. Accept help with your other responsibilities.

- Try not to share your baby too much during this time – you can easily miss feeding cues if someone else is holding him.

- Encourage your baby to feed frequently in the first couple of weeks, to set your breasts up for maximum milk production, help you avoid engorgement, and give you both plenty of practice.

- Hold your baby skin to skin whenever you can and keep him near you day and night.

- Avoid giving your baby formula or water unless there are medical reasons why he needs them – at least for the first two weeks but preferably for the first six months.

- Avoid giving your baby a dummy or feeding him with a bottle – at least for the first two weeks.

- Get to know your breasts and how they feel now they're 'working'.

- Learn to express your milk by hand.

6

Knowing it's working

'The problem with breastfeeding is that you can't see how much the baby is getting.' This is a familiar lament. Many women worry about whether or not their baby is having enough milk, especially in the early weeks. Breastfeeding babies regulate their own appetites, so the only person who really knows whether she's getting enough milk is your baby. Part of baby-led breastfeeding involves learning to recognise the everyday signs that will tell you how well breastfeeding is going – from your point of view and your baby's. This chapter shows you how.

Knowing what to look for

For many decades most people in the UK – including health professionals – have been more familiar with formula feeding than they are with breastfeeding. The behaviour of formula-fed babies (regular feeds with long periods of sleep), together with their average intake of milk (which can be measured exactly), have been used as benchmarks for judging whether or not a baby is getting enough.

The parent-led nature of formula feeding has made us wary of trusting babies to decide for themselves how often to feed and how long to feed for – especially when we can't see how much milk they're taking. So when a baby has an erratic pattern, with frequent feeds of varying lengths (perfectly normal for a breastfed baby), it's easy to assume that something is wrong.

> 'I was baffled by the irregularity of Kyla's feeds in the early weeks – especially when she wanted lots of feeds in the evening. I was convinced feeds should be evenly spaced out and I'd get really worried that she didn't have a pattern. But she did – it just wasn't the one I thought she should have.'
>
> *Eva, mother of Kyla, seven months*

Breastfed babies naturally feed at different rates, so watching the clock won't tell you how much milk your baby is taking. In general, babies get faster at feeding as they mature but, even then, the same baby can choose to spin out some feeds and race through others (even if she takes the same amount of milk each time) – just as you do with your meals. Breastmilk also varies between mothers and throughout the day (see page 29). All of this means that it's impossible to measure how much milk your baby is taking – or even to know exactly how much she needs. But you don't need to: your baby is the one who makes these decisions. What you *can* do is work out if what she's getting is enough to keep her healthy and help her grow – and there are lots of signs you can look for:

- Watching and listening to your baby while she's feeding will tell you whether she's taking plenty of milk at *this* feed.
- How your breasts feel and look immediately after a feed will tell you what happened during that feed (as well as helping you to spot signs of infection or other problems).
- Your baby's wees and poos will tell you what's been happening over the last few hours.
- Your baby's behaviour, weight and general appearance will tell you what's been happening over the last few days.

Watching and listening to your baby feed

Breastfed babies have a typical pattern of sucking and swallowing during feeds. How well your baby fits this pattern at each feed – and how she ends the feed – will reveal a lot about whether she's getting lots of milk.

What happens at the beginning of the feed

Most babies will attach to the breast fairly quickly as long as they are calm, ready to feed and can scoop up a good mouthful easily. Some babies come on and off the breast several times before they start to suck, as they work to get the nipple into the most comfortable place. Unless your baby is lying on top of you (in which case she can adjust her position herself), you may need to be ready to modify the way you're holding her, to make it easier for her to get the right angle.

A baby who persistently attaches and lets go at the start of a feed *may* have a tongue tie (see page 40) which is making it difficult for her to attach effectively. If she comes off the breast crying after a few sucks or doesn't seem to want to go near it at all, the problem could be 'breast refusal', which has many possible causes (see *If your baby goes on strike*, page 124). Remember that a baby who has had to wait to feed and has been crying may simply be finding it difficult to calm down enough to latch on – or she may have a tummy full of wind (see page 81).

Watching and listening for sucking and swallowing

Your baby's pattern of sucking and swallowing can give you a good idea how much milk she is taking during a feed. In the first couple of days, while she is getting mainly colostrum, she may not swallow very often. However, from the third day onwards you should be able to see (or hear) her sucking and swallowing in this sort of pattern:

- At the beginning of the feed there will probably be a burst of short, rapid sucks with little or no swallowing. This could last a second or two or it could last a few minutes. During this time your baby is making sure she has your nipple a long way back in her mouth and is waiting for your let-down reflex to work.

- Once your milk is flowing, as long as she is effectively attached your baby will relax and settle down to a pattern of big yawning sucks (see page 32) and swallows – usually one or two 'yawns' to each swallow. This rhythm tells you that she is getting a big mouthful of milk with each suck. Some babies swallow very loudly. Others do it almost silently, with just a little outward breath (like a quick puff of air) from their nose after each one. Sometimes it's easier to see a baby swallow than to hear her. If your baby is swallowing, she's getting milk.

- If your baby wants just a small drink she will stop feeding quite quickly. If not, she'll carry on in short bursts of 'yawns' and swallows, with occasional pauses for a rest.

- After a while, as the milk gets gradually thicker and creamier (see page 29), the flow will start to slow down and you'll notice her swallowing less frequently.

- As your baby gets ready to come off the breast her pauses will get longer and she'll do very little swallowing. She may look as though she is falling asleep. Her chin may quiver slightly, followed by a short flurry of quick sucks (called 'flutter sucking'), and another long pause. It's tempting to assume, when you see this, that she is just sucking for comfort and that you should take her off the breast but this is when your milk is at its creamiest. She's still getting food – in small amounts but packed full of calories. She will come off by herself – but not quite yet.

- When she lets go, she may want to continue her feed on your other breast, either straight away or after a rest, taking just a few sucks or going through the whole cycle again, depending on her hunger.

This pattern is very different from that of a baby feeding from a bottle, whose suck-swallow rhythm stays more or less the same throughout the feed. Bottle feeding is more tiring for babies as they have to pause frequently to take a breath, whereas a breastfeeding baby can breathe while she sucks.

Your baby will end the feed

Babies *always* come off the breast by themselves when they've had enough milk. If they don't, they haven't. Typically, the baby's sucking will slow down as she reaches the creamiest milk near the end of the feed (see above), until eventually she pushes the nipple out with her tongue. She may smack her lips and have a satisfied 'drunk' look on her face – like the baby in photo number 7.

Babies often fall asleep at the breast. This is the most natural thing in the world, but it can occasionally be a sign that breastfeeding is not going well. A baby who is ineffectively attached has to work hard to get milk and may fall asleep because she's exhausted. Unlike the baby who's had enough milk (who will usually stay asleep), she'll often wake up as the nipple falls out of her mouth and want to go straight back on again, because she didn't mean to let go and her tummy isn't full.

A breastfeed can be as short as a few sucks or as long as three-quarters of an hour. And a baby can feed from just one breast or both – or even go from one to the other several times. Only your baby knows what she needs at that particular feed and only she knows when she's had it. But if she consistently wants to feed for longer than about 45 minutes,

USING BREASTFEEDING TO SETTLE YOUR BABY

For a baby, breastfeeding is comforting and soothing – a lovely way to drift off to sleep. Allowing your baby to relax and let go of the breast in her own time is a good thing, not a bad one. She will gradually find ways to settle herself and fall asleep on her own but she doesn't need to be deprived of her main source of comfort in order to do that.

or falls asleep at the breast and is awake again 10 minutes later, it's worth checking her attachment.

If it hurts, it's not right

Painful breastfeeding – even in the first few weeks – is a sign that something is wrong. And even if your baby *seems* to be feeding well, if it's hurting you it's probably not right for her either.

Your nipples may be slightly sensitive in the first few days – a few seconds of 'ouch' at the beginning of a feed isn't unusual (see page 38). But that's all. After that, the feed should be pain free. Mostly, the reason for painful breastfeeding is that the baby isn't attached effectively, which means she won't be getting as much milk as she should. Occasionally it's caused by an infection. Either way, it needs attention quickly, so if you can't fix it yourself (see *Painful breastfeeding: quick symptom checker*, page 275), you will need to get some help.

When your baby comes off your breast it's a good idea to check that your nipple is the same shape and colour as it was before it went in. It may look a bit longer, because it's been slightly stretched, but it shouldn't look pinched or wedge-shaped, or be white or blue (see page 229). If it *is* an odd shape or colour, it's probably been squashed against the hard part of the roof of her mouth or between her gums, indicating that she hasn't taken in a big enough mouthful of breast.

Feeling your breasts for lumps and bumps occasionally (maybe once a day, after a feed) is a good way to make sure you pick up problems such as blocked ducts early, so you can deal with them before they become painful. See *Painful breast-feeding: quick symptom checker*, page 275 for what to do if you find something unusual.

Signs that your baby is feeding effectively

- Her body is relaxed, not tense, while she's feeding.
- She feeds rhythmically, with slow, deep sucks and occasional pauses.
- She swallows after every one or two sucks for most of the feed.
- The pauses get gradually longer and the swallows less frequent.
- She pushes or spits your nipple out of her mouth and looks satisfied.
- Your nipples are the same shape and colour after the feed as they were before.
- Feeding doesn't hurt and your nipples and breasts aren't sore.

Signs that need attention

- Your baby comes on and off the breast during a feed.
- Her sucking is shallow and erratic rather than deep and rhythmic.
- She swallows only after every three or more sucks.
- She never takes herself off the breast, or she falls off then wants to feed again immediately.
- One or both of your nipples is an odd shape or colour when it comes out of your baby's mouth.
- One or both of your nipples hurts all the time your baby is feeding, or is cracked or bleeding.
- Your breasts are sore, painful, lumpy or inflamed.

Wees and poos – the best clues

One of the best ways to tell whether your baby is getting enough milk is to check her wees and poos. If there's enough going in, there will be plenty coming out.

Wees are the best guide to how much milk your baby has had in the last 6 to 12 hours. Poos (together with wees) are the best guide to how much milk your baby has had in the last 24 hours. (This assumes she is having only your milk. If she is being given anything else – even water – her wees and poos won't give a reliable picture.)

> 'I had no confidence when I came home from hospital. I was convinced I didn't have enough milk. Olivia wanted to be on the breast all the time so I thought she must be starving. I made notes of all her feeds to show the health visitor. Eventually I realised it was normal for her to feed that much and that I could easily tell by her nappies that she was getting enough milk.'
>
> *Kate, mother of Olivia, five months*

How often should my baby do a wee?

Babies don't need to drink much for the first few days and the early milk (colostrum) is very concentrated, so breastfed babies don't pass a lot of urine during this time. But if they are feeding well their output will build up quickly as they

---

PINK WEE

Sometimes the nappy of a newborn baby contains pinkish or orangey spots. These are urate crystals, which occasionally form in concentrated urine. This is quite normal and doesn't usually last more than a day or two because, as milk production gets going, the baby will be drinking more.

start to take in more milk. A good guide for the first five days is to expect *at least* one wee on the first day, two on the second, three on the third, and so on. After this, your baby should be producing at least six pale yellow wees every day. If her milk intake suddenly goes up or down, you will notice a change in her wees within a few hours.

Urine doesn't show up very well in some nappies (especially the disposable type) so the best guide is how heavy the nappy is. Pouring 45ml of water into a dry nappy will give you an idea of how it should feel.

What should my baby's poos look like?

Changes in your baby's poo in the first five days will show you how well she is feeding. The first stool is meconium, which is very thick, sticky, and black or greeny-black in colour. You can expect your baby to pass meconium two or three times before the colour starts to change. (Some babies pass meconium during labour as well.)

Some time between 24 and 48 hours after the birth you will probably notice the poo becoming slightly less sticky and more yellowy-green in colour. This is known as a 'changing stool' and it's a sign that milk has begun to work its way through your baby's digestive system. It will then get progressively more orangey-yellow in colour and more runny, until, by day four or five, it's like korma sauce or runny yellow mustard. Photos number 8 to 10 show what you can expect your baby's poo to look like over the first five days.

The amount of poo is more variable than for wees but from her second day onwards your baby should be producing *at least* two teaspoonful-sized poos (or larger) per day. If she isn't producing runny yellow poos by her fifth day, it's likely that she hasn't been getting all the milk she should. In that case, ask your midwife or a breastfeeding supporter to check her feeding technique and see if they can suggest some adjustments (see *Where can I get help?*, page 106).

Wees and poos in the first five days

Day after birth	Wee		Poo	
	Appearance	How many times in 24 hours?	Appearance	How many times in 24 hours?
1st	Pale yellow. May contain pinkish spots.	At least 1	Thick, sticky, greeny-black	At least 1
2nd	Pale yellow	At least 2	Less sticky; more yellowy-green ('changing stool')	At least 2
3rd	Pale yellow	At least 3	Runnier and more yellow	At least 2; probably 3 or more
4th	Pale yellow	At least 4	Runnier and more orangey-yellow	At least 2; probably 4 or more
5th	Pale yellow	At least 5	Runny; orangey-yellow (like korma sauce or yellow mustard)	At least 2; probably 5 or more
After this	Pale yellow	At least 6	Runny; orangey-yellow (like korma sauce or yellow mustard)	At least 2; probably 6 or more (until at least 4 weeks)

Your baby should continue to produce at least two poos (and probably more) per day for the first four to six weeks. After this, her stools may suddenly become less frequent and she may go for several days (maybe even a week or more) without producing a poo at all. This is quite normal – but *not* in the first few weeks. If it happens then, it suggests she isn't taking in enough milk.

The colour of your baby's poo may vary a bit between orange and green, but mostly it will stay yellow (and runny) all the time she is on breastmilk alone. It may appear to have 'seeds' in it sometimes; this is normal. People who are used to the darker, more solid poo of a formula-fed baby sometimes think that breastmilk must be 'going straight through', or that the baby has diarrhoea. But it's this yellow, runny, slightly sweet-smelling type of poo that babies are supposed to produce. (See *What to expect when* on page 271 for a quick summary.)

> 'I couldn't believe how much poo Ethan produced. After a few weeks he stopped going so often – he just used to save it up and then there'd be a massive explosion – up to his neck and down to his knees! At least it didn't smell bad.'
>
> Chantelle, mother of Ethan, 10 months

Your baby's behaviour can tell you a lot

Your baby's feeding pattern will be unique and no two days will be exactly the same. But how she behaves between feeds and when she comes to the breast can tell you a lot about how breastfeeding is going.

The too-contented baby

Most babies who aren't getting enough milk let their parents know, by asking vigorously for feeds and crying a lot. But some babies don't have enough energy to do this, either because they haven't been getting much milk for quite a while or because they are ill. They may show only fleeting feeding cues and sleep most of the time – and the fact that something is wrong can easily go unnoticed.

Babies are not supposed to feed infrequently and sleep for long periods. They should have periods of alertness, when they are looking around and wanting to be talked to. And they should want to feed often. If your baby is asking for feeds fewer than six times in 24 hours (eight times every 24 hours in the first two weeks) and sleeping almost all the time – especially if she is jaundiced (see page 84) – look carefully at her behaviour during feeds and check her wees and poos. If in doubt, seek help (see *Where can I get help?*, page 106).

Expecting a baby to feed infrequently and to spend much of the day on her own or sleeping (often referred to as being 'contented') is not realistic or safe – and it's not good for breastfeeding.

The 'colicky' baby

Babies who cry a lot are often said to have 'colic'. It tends to be more common in the evenings and is thought by many people to indicate tummy-ache. However, it's not always clear that the problem really *is* tummy-ache. Many 'colicky' babies settle down if they are held or offered a feed, suggesting that they were just hungry or needing extra reassurance. Some babies who are diagnosed with 'evening colic' simply need to feed a lot in the evenings (see *Babies like to feed in clusters*, page 111); not responding to them when they ask makes them distressed. And babies who have to wait to be fed can be colicky because they've swallowed air while crying. However, if your baby is colicky and none of the above scenarios applies, the problem could be 'breastfeeding colic'.

A baby who has breastfeeding colic usually cries (or screams) for long periods soon after a feed. She is difficult to console, often drawing her knees up towards her chest or arching her back. Her poo is likely to be quite distinctive – greenish, watery-looking, maybe even frothy – and there's lots of it.

Babies with breastfeeding colic tend to want to feed very frequently and some don't gain weight as they should. Because of this, mothers whose babies are colicky are sometimes told that their milk isn't rich enough for their baby, or that it doesn't suit her. This isn't true – there's nothing wrong with the milk. The answer lies in the feeding.

There are two main reasons for breastfeeding colic:

- The baby is not feeding effectively.
- The baby is not able to feed for long enough.

Either of these will mean your baby will tend to get the watery – and sugary – 'soup course' but she won't get as far as the creamy, fat-laden 'dessert', which is an essential part of the feed. So she ends up with too much sugar compared with the amount of fat. This causes the milk to rush through the gut without being fully digested, giving the poo its green colour and watery consistency. The excess sugar ferments, producing gas, which causes pain. The combination of an irritated gut and lots of gas results in 'explosive' stools that are passed fast and noisily and a baby who is miserable.

If your baby has the symptoms of breastfeeding colic, have a careful look at the way she is feeding. Make sure she gets a good mouthful of breast (see page 32), and let her feed for as long as she wants. This will mean she'll get all the fat she should. You'll probably notice a difference in her behaviour and her poo within 24 hours – possibly sooner. In the meantime, holding her in an upright position or giving her a gentle massage or some skin-to-skin time may help to make her more comfortable.

A less common cause of colic occurring after the first few weeks is that the mother is producing excessive amounts of milk, so her baby gets too much of the thinner milk and has no room for the creamier milk (see *Could I be making too much milk?*, page 212). Occasionally it can be the result of something the mother has eaten (see page 130). Rarely, colicky behaviour is a sign of a more serious condition, such as reflux disease (see page 82). If you can't identify the cause of your baby's crying, ask your doctor to check her over.

'My grandma and my friends were pressuring me to bottle feed because Tom was so colicky – they kept saying I didn't have enough milk. But I just *knew* he wasn't hungry. Eventually I saw a breastfeeding supporter and she explained I'd been taking him off the breast too soon. I thought he'd fallen asleep when he was still going. Once I stopped doing that he was fine – and much happier.'

Becky, mother of Tom, nine months

If your baby refuses to feed

If your baby refuses the breast, crying loudly and arching her back to avoid it, it can be distressing for both of you. While your nurturing instinct is telling you to hold her close, she seems to be pushing you away.

The most common cause of breast refusal in a young baby is that the baby has been repeatedly held in an uncomfortable or awkward position for feeding. This makes breastfeeding unpleasant and frustrating for her, and she will associate the breast with these feelings. It's very difficult for a baby to breast-feed if she can't tilt her head back, or if she has to twist her head sideways to get to the breast. She'll struggle to open her mouth wide enough to feed and it will be difficult for her to swallow.

If you think your baby's position could be the problem, try adjusting the way you hold her so that she can feed more easily. Lying back with her on your tummy (see page 43) will allow her to feed with the minimum of handling and may help you both to get your confidence back. If this doesn't solve the problem it may be that you need to concentrate on helping her to feel happy near your breast again, and to get back to her instincts for breastfeeding. The way to do this is described on page 126.

Occasionally babies refuse the breast if it tastes or smells strange to them. This can happen when the mother uses scented wipes or soap on her nipples before feeding. There's no need to clean your nipples before you feed your baby.

If your baby is happy to feed for a minute or two and *then* pulls away, it could be that the milk flow is too fast for her, especially if she comes off spluttering. This is most likely to happen at the beginning of the feed, when the let-down reflex is strongest. See page 80 for how to deal with this. Rarely, breast refusal is a sign of reflux disease (see page 82).

Occasionally, feeding is painful for a newborn baby because her skull bones are slightly out of alignment following the birth. Some parents have found that cranial osteopathy, in which the skull is gently manipulated back into shape, is helpful in these circumstances. If you can't find an obvious answer for your baby's refusal to feed you may want to seek out a registered osteopath who specialises in cranial work and who is used to treating babies (see *Sources of information and support*, page 278).

In a baby older than one month, a sudden episode of breast refusal (also called a nursing strike) is more likely to be caused by something unconnected with the feeding itself. See page 124 for some possible causes, and tips on what to do.

What to expect with your baby's weight

Many parents and health professionals put a lot of emphasis on a baby's weight and, as they grow, many babies are weighed much more often than they need to be. Weight *is* important but it's not enough on its own to tell you whether breastfeeding is going well – and it's a fairly slow way of spotting feeding problems.

Weight gain in the early days

It's normal for babies to lose a small amount of weight in the first few days. However, they shouldn't lose very much, and they will usually begin to gain weight again on about their fourth day, as milk production gets going. Excessive weight loss – 10 per cent or more – in the first few days can be a sign of illness but more often it's an indication that the baby hasn't been getting enough milk.

Your baby's weight gain is related to how much milk she takes in. If she doesn't get the milk you are making she won't thrive – and your breasts will start to cut down production (see *Production on demand – how it works*, page 25). However, weight gain (or loss) doesn't tell you what's happening *now* with your baby's feeds, only what has happened over the past few days. Your baby's feeding behaviour and her wees and poos are a much more immediate guide (see above). If you ignore these signs and wait to see how much weight she has gained, your milk production may slow down in the meantime, giving you a double problem (still solvable, but not quite as easily).

If your baby is healthy, feeding effectively and weeing and pooing normally, then (except in the first couple of days) she *will* be gaining weight. If her feeding technique, wees and poos are all okay and she *isn't* gaining weight, then something else is wrong and she should be investigated for illness.

How often should I weigh my baby?

Babies tend to gain weight in fits and starts, rather than constantly. While she shouldn't *lose* weight after the first few days, or stay the same weight for very long at a time, there is no reason to expect your baby to put on weight at a steady rate, week after week, so there's no advantage in weighing her frequently. A couple of weighings in the first two weeks is a good idea, just to make sure she is adjusting well to life outside the womb. After that, unless there are particular concerns about her health, there's no need to weigh her more than once a month. Every two months is fine after she reaches six months and, if you want to carry on having her weighed once she reaches a year, every three to six months is plenty.

What if it's not working?

When breastfeeding goes wrong, the answer usually lies in going back to the basics. If you suspect that breastfeeding isn't going well, for either you or for your baby, start by looking at her feeding pattern over a 24-hour period and watching her closely while she's feeding. A quiet day or two with plenty of skin-to-skin contact may be enough to put things right. Have another look at Chapters 3 and 5, to remind you what to look for and how to make sure feeding is effective. If you can't find the answer – or are struggling to change things – get some help.

Where can I get help?

Although a midwife, health visitor or GP is the most obvious person to turn to when you are concerned about your baby's feeding, not all health professionals have had in-depth training on breastfeeding so they may not necessarily be the best people to help. In the UK, some NHS trusts employ specialist breastfeeding supporters, who run clinics and may even do home visits, but in most areas this type of help is provided by volunteer breastfeeding supporters (sometimes called breastfeeding counsellors), via support groups and telephone helplines (see *Getting support from other mothers*, page 121). BabyCafe™ drop-ins are run jointly by volunteer supporters and health professionals. There are also independent lactation consultants (who normally charge for their services) and there are several websites that provide helpful breastfeeding information (see *Sources of information and support*, page 278).

Key points

- Watching and listening to your baby as she feeds will tell you whether she's getting milk. Look for a rhythm of big yawning sucks with frequent swallows that gradually slows down as the milk gets creamier.

- If your baby goes on and off the breast at the start of the feed she's probably finding it difficult to attach.

- If your baby doesn't come off the breast by herself, or if she almost always feeds for more than 45 minutes, then she's probably struggling to get milk.

- Checking your nipples for damage after feeds, and your breasts for lumps and inflammation once a day, will help you to spot feeding problems early.

- Wees and poos are the best clues to whether your baby is getting enough milk.

- Babies under four weeks should poo at *least* twice a day; older babies may go several days without a poo.

- If your baby is miserable, feeds very frequently and has green poo, check the way she's feeding.

- If a young baby refuses the breast, the most likely reason is that she is being held awkwardly.

- If your baby is sleepy and not asking for many feeds, seek help.

- Weight isn't the best way to check how breastfeeding is going – other signs are more helpful.

- If you have any doubts about how breastfeeding is going, seek help. The earlier you find out what's wrong, the easier it will be to fix it.

7

Settling in to breastfeeding

As you follow your baby's lead, the intensity of the first few weeks of breastfeeding will gradually lessen. Your baby will develop a more predictable rhythm and, as you both gain experience, you'll start to feel that you don't need to concentrate so much each time he feeds. This chapter is about the changes you can expect over the next few months, how to adjust to your baby's natural patterns of feeding and why trying to get him into a routine is unlikely to work. (For an overview of what to expect throughout the time your baby is breastfeeding, see *What to expect when*, page 271.)

Getting breastfeeding 'established'

Technically, it takes about six weeks for milk production to 'become established' – that is, for a mother's breasts to work out a pattern of milk production that suits her baby. But after two or three weeks you'll probably notice that your breasts feel less full between feeds, they leak less often and your let-down reflex is more reliable.

Establishing *breastfeeding* is slightly different. It's about you and your baby learning to work together so that feeding is second nature, instead of something you have to concentrate on. It's about reaching the stage when you don't notice how many times your baby feeds over the course of the day and through the night, as you and he respond more intuitively to each other and feeding is less effort.

How long it will take for you and your baby to reach this level of confidence is difficult to predict. Even if you've breastfed a baby before, this new relationship will be different. Some mothers and babies are confident after a week or two; others can take a couple of months. You probably won't know until you look back and realise things suddenly feel much easier. The key is to give yourself and your baby plenty of time and opportunities to practise, and to trust each other.

Why routines don't work

Attempting to impose your own schedule – or one from a book – is likely to disrupt breastfeeding. Most adult-designed routines are based on set times for feeding and sleeping (and sometimes even for playing). Usually there are quite long gaps between feeds. Breastfeeding isn't designed to work like this.

Breastfeeding is more than food and drink – it also provides babies with comfort, company, warmth and security. None of these things can be regulated by the clock, so expecting your baby to fit into a schedule is unrealistic. For a mother, in the short term controlling or restricting feeding is likely to lead to engorgement (see page 285); in the longer term it will cause less milk to be made. If you are one of the rare women who naturally over-produce milk it's possible such a routine will work for *you* – but it probably won't work for your baby.

It's unlikely babies have any concept of the future. Their survival instincts tell them their need is urgent and research suggests that if they don't get a quick response they feel frightened. Trying to fight your baby's instincts to be fed and held will make him – and you – stressed and miserable. Responding to his needs promptly will make life easier for both of you. It's not about allowing your baby to rule your life; it's about adjusting your life to include your baby.

Your baby will eventually eat and sleep at conventional times, but not yet. In the meantime, making an active decision to let him lead the way will make breastfeeding – and parenting – much easier than trying to force things into a routine. Many families who start by trying to establish a routine quickly discover that keeping their baby near and responding to his needs is better for breastfeeding – and for family life generally.

'The unpredictability of everything made me panicky in the first few months, so I started following a routine from a book, with three-hourly feeds, times to sleep, play and have "me-time". I thought the structure would make me feel better but I ended up pacing round with Emily screaming, waiting for the three hours to be up. Even if *I* wanted a routine, it wasn't working for her – she was miserable. Eventually I realised a happy baby meant a happy mum. It had to be that way round – because no one is happy if the baby is screaming.'

Julie, mother of Emily, 18 months

Your baby's changing patterns

For the first few weeks your baby's feeds will probably be unpredictable, and life may feel quite chaotic. After that, although no two days will be exactly the same, you'll start to see a pattern emerging. He may start to feed slightly less often at night, especially if he is able to feed frequently in the evenings. During the day, his appetite will vary (like yours), with some feeds very short and some quite long. He'll almost certainly continue to want at least six feeds in 24 hours – and probably many more – though it's unlikely you'll feel the need to count them.

'I thought I was feeding on demand until I went to a baby group and I saw a woman *really* feeding on demand. I had no idea how she knew her baby needed a feed but she'd be chatting away to someone and every now and then, almost without looking, she'd just lift him to her breast and he'd have a little feed. She seemed completely in tune with him.'

Kim, mother of Sadie, six months

Babies like to feed in clusters

Many babies want lots of feeds close together, in batches or 'clusters', especially in the evenings. They can get very distressed if their need for feeding isn't met, and this unsettled behaviour and crying is often mistaken for colic (see page 101).

The constant on-off nature of cluster feeding can make ordinary tasks such as cooking a meal or washing up difficult. Getting to know your baby's individual pattern will make it easier for you to plan for this (for example, by preparing some of the meal in advance, using a slow cooker, or sharing the cooking with your partner).

Working out how to feed your baby in a sling can also help with cluster feeding, because it allows you to have your hands free to get on with other things, even if your baby is on and off the breast all evening. If there's nothing else you need to be doing, lying back on the sofa with your baby on top of you, so he can latch on whenever he needs to, may be the easiest solution. That way *he* won't have to keep asking and *you* won't have to keep picking him up and rearranging your clothes.

Many (though not all) babies who develop a pattern of evening cluster feeding have a longer period of sleep afterwards. Resisting your baby's requests for feeding is likely to make him unsettled all evening – and most of the night as well – whereas if you give in to what's happening and let him feed on and off throughout the evening you're likely to get more sleep.

'I wasted a lot of time and energy trying to fit my first baby's feeds into a pattern that worked for me but not for him. Once I resigned myself to sitting on the sofa all evening and stopped trying to put my boobs away, it all seemed to get easier. I didn't make the same mistake with the next two when they wanted to feed all evening. I just read a book or watched TV while they fed.'

*Margaret, mother of Paul, ten years, James, nine years,
and Lisa, seven years*

Expect appetite spurts

Sometimes a baby will suddenly start to feed more frequently than usual and then settle back to a familiar feeding pattern after a few days. This is called an 'appetite spurt' (or a 'growth spurt' or 'hunger spurt'). It happens because the baby is feeling extra hungry and needs to stimulate more milk (although it doesn't necessarily coincide with him growing faster than usual). A few days of increased feeding is all that's needed to give the breasts the message that they need to make more.

YOU DON'T ALWAYS HAVE TO WAIT FOR YOUR BABY TO ASK

Feeding your baby whenever he wants may make you wonder if you'll ever be able to plan anything. But you don't have to wait for him to ask every time. Most young babies are open to breastfeeding whenever they're awake – and sometimes even when they're not! If you need to nip out somewhere – or start a long journey – and don't want to risk your baby wanting a feed the minute you set foot outside the door, you can offer him the opportunity to feed *before* he asks. If he's asleep, just rubbing his nose gently against your nipple or expressing a few drops of milk on to his lips may be enough to tempt him to at least have a quick snack.

Feeding at night

Night feeds are important. Babies aren't born knowing that their parents have designated night-time as sleep time. Most babies feed more frequently in the evening and early part of the night (7pm–3am) than they do in the early morning and during the day (3am–7pm), for at least the first few weeks. Feeding as often as your baby needs, night and day, is the best way to ensure you make plenty of milk and avoid engorgement (see page 235). Breastfeeding relies on you and your baby staying in sync 24 hours a day.

'It took me a long time to respond to Lilly instinctively during the day. There were so many distractions and I was a bit stressed. It was different at night. It's a different kind of sleep with a baby. I'd be asleep but also very aware of her movements, and I'd always wake up to feed just before she stirred. I was much more in tune with her – it felt more instinctive and intimate.'

Hannah, mother of Lilly, 10 months

Pressure to get a baby to sleep all night can often come from people who think babies should be 'taught' to manage on their own, or who are used to formula feeding, which tends to be less frequent. But babies are not supposed to sleep too deeply; they're meant to wake frequently to feed. Night feeds are easier if you don't *expect* your baby to sleep right through.

'My mum was always asking if Nathan was sleeping through yet. So we just decided "night" meant midnight to 5am. That way we could tell her that Nathan only woke once! It took a bit of the pressure off.'

Kieran, father of Nathan, three months

Here are some tips for making feeding at night easier to manage:

- Go to bed early if you can.
- Offer your baby a feed immediately before you go to bed. There's no need to wake him – just hold him next to your breast and talk to him gently, or express some milk on to his lips to encourage him to latch on.
- Keep your baby in the same room with you – or, if it's safe (see box below), in your bed. This will help to co-ordinate your sleep cycle with his, so that you're already waking up when he starts to stir and can feed him without either of you needing to wake up fully. (An alternative to bed sharing is a three-sided 'arm's reach' or 'co-sleeper' cot that clips on to your bed, allowing you to reach your baby easily.)
- Offer your baby a feed as soon as he begins to wake, before he starts to cry.
- Learn to feed lying down, so you can rest while your baby feeds.
- Sleep naked, or wear an easy-to-open nightdress, pyjama top or bra. (If you tend to leak milk, spread a thick towel underneath your top half, to protect the bed.)
- Learn to feed in the dark, so you don't have to wake everybody up by switching on the light. (And so your baby doesn't start to associate darkness with being hungry or lonely and light with food and comfort.) Practise during the day by feeding with your eyes shut.
- Don't change your baby's nappy at night unless it's very wet, he's done a poo, or he's got a nappy rash.
- Have a drink nearby in case you are thirsty.
- Help your baby to decide to do more of his feeding during the day by making a point of not tip-toeing around him in the mornings – even if you're grateful that he's finally gone to sleep!

- Snatch 40 winks whenever you can while your baby is asleep during the day.

Bed sharing and co-sleeping

Sharing your bed with your baby can make night-time feeding easier, which is probably why mothers who sleep with their babies tend to breastfeed for longer than those who don't. However, you need to be sure he's safe, so:

- Make sure he isn't overdressed and there's nothing that could cover his head. The risk of overheating comes from your baby's clothes and the bedclothes, which will tend to prevent him losing heat, not from your body, which will usually help regulate his temperature.
- If there is another child in the bed, make sure an adult sleeps between the child and the baby.
- Sleep on your side, curled round your baby, with his head at the level of your breast. This makes feeding easier, keeps him from going into the pillows or being lain on and lets him roll on to his back to sleep when he lets go of your breast.
- Don't leave your baby alone in your bed.

Bed sharing is NOT a good idea if:
- There is any way your baby could get trapped or injured, either in the bed or by falling out of it.
- Either you or your partner is a smoker.
- Either you or your partner might not be able to respond normally to your baby (for example, if you are ill, or you have drunk alcohol or taken a drug or medicine which could make you sleep unusually deeply).
- You have a saggy mattress or a waterbed, which could cause your baby to end up in a dip.

- Your baby was born early and has not yet reached his due date, or he is ill (meaning that he may not be able to alert you if he is in trouble).
- There are pets in or on the bed.

Even if you don't plan for your baby to stay in your bed after his feeds, it's best to make sure the environment is safe, just in case you fall asleep.

NB: **Sleeping with your baby in an armchair or on a sofa is very dangerous.** Babies can wriggle or fall into gaps or under cushions and become wedged or covered. If you feel tired and want to lie down to feed during the day, your bed is a safer place than the sofa.

'I couldn't believe how much more sleep I got when I started lying down to feed and letting Rhian stay in the bed. For the first eight weeks I'd sit upright to feed at night and then insist on putting her back in the cot. It was counter-productive because it meant we were both awake and unsettled for longer. I had to wake up properly for each feed and she never wanted to go back in the cot, so she was always hard to settle. I think I would have died of tiredness if I hadn't figured it out.'

Amy, *mother of Rhian, 14 months*

Why a bottle isn't the answer

Partners are often encouraged to help new mothers by doing 'the night feed'. This is a great way for parents to share the care of a bottle-fed baby but taking over a night feed for a breastfeeding mother is *not* helpful and can lead to all sorts of extra problems, especially if the baby is given formula. Here's why:

- Replacing a breastfeed with a bottle will affect your milk production. Cutting out night-time breastfeeds can mean you don't produce enough milk for your baby.
- Missing a breastfeed can lead to engorgement, and possibly even mastitis (see Chapter 13). This is a risk even if the replacement feed is previously expressed breastmilk.
- If your baby is still learning to breastfeed, giving him a bottle may mean he struggles to latch on next time, leading to an increased risk of soreness for you and frustration for you both.
- If your baby is starting to have a longer period of sleep at night, replacing a feed at the beginning or end of it could lead to a very long gap between breastfeeds, increasing the risk of problems still further.

Some parents switch to formula in the hope of getting more sleep only to find that, although feeding happens less often, it tends to be more disruptive and tiring. Or they discover that their baby wasn't waking because he was hungry – he just needed comfort and reassurance. Without breastfeeding they have to find another way to soothe him back to sleep. And without breastfeeding, getting back to sleep may be harder for you, too. So although it may be tempting to give a bottle at night, providing your baby is right next to you you'll probably find it's easier to breastfeed.

Breastfeeding when you're out and about

One of the advantages of breastmilk is that's it's the perfect 'fast food' for your baby: you always have it ready at the right temperature, so you can spend time away from home without having to plan for feeds. This makes going out and travelling much easier. However, it's common to feel uneasy about breastfeeding when there are other people around, especially the first time.

Feeding in public doesn't mean you have to expose your breasts. Many mothers breastfeed in shops, cafés and on trains and buses without anyone being aware of what they are doing. If you think you might be embarrassed, there are plenty of things you can do to make feeding discreet – both in advance and at the time.

Having a babymoon (see page 68) provides a great opportunity to get the hang of breastfeeding without anyone watching you. Practising undoing a breastfeeding bra with one hand and feeding with your eyes closed can help you to do it by feel. It's also worth experimenting with alternative ways of holding your baby for feeding (see Chapter 3) and with different types of clothes (see page 18). **If you're nervous about how much flesh people might see, try feeding in front of a mirror (or your partner or a friend); most women are surprised to realise how little is revealed.**

Once you and your baby have had plenty of practice (and he has developed better control of his head and neck) he'll be able to latch on quickly and you won't have to look at what he's doing or fumble with your clothes. You'll be able to feed your baby with him tucked out of sight inside your (loose) T-shirt or jumper, under a shawl or muslin or in a sling. (It's worth checking that whatever you are wearing will be easy to feed in before you leave the house – lifting up a dress can be awkward!)

It may help to be with someone else the first time you go out with your baby, and to find a quiet spot to feed in case he takes a while to latch on. You may want to choose a café or restaurant that is popular with mothers and babies – the staff will probably be used to seeing breastfeeding and there may be other mothers feeding while you are there.

As your baby gets older and becomes increasingly interested in what's going on around him he is likely to come off the breast now and then while he's feeding – perhaps to smile at you, or to watch other people. If you don't want anyone to see your breast when this happens you'll need to move your

T-shirt quickly, or grab a muslin to cover up. He may want to play with your clothes or stroke your other breast. If this bothers you, try giving him something else to play with (a necklace can work well) or gently holding his hand as he feeds.

Although there are occasionally stories in the press about mothers being asked to stop breastfeeding, in reality this is very rare. **In the UK, it is an offence for anyone to prevent a mother from breastfeeding her baby in a public place.** (In Scotland, mothers are legally guaranteed this protection until their child is two years old.)

Nowadays, lots of areas have 'breastfeeding welcome' initiatives. Local shops, cafés, sports centres and public buildings display a sticker or poster to show mothers that they are especially welcome to breastfeed on the premises. You can find details online (see page 281), or find out from your midwife, health visitor or local breastfeeding group whether there is a scheme in your area.

'I had to feed Phoebe the other night in a restaurant with my in-laws. They said: "Can't you wait till you get home?" But they were absolutely fine about it once they realised nobody could actually see anything. And I really didn't want to carry a screaming baby all the way home just to feed her.'

Andrea, mother of Ryan, four years, and Phoebe, one year

Getting support from other people

Looking after a mother during the first few weeks, so she can concentrate on her baby and on breastfeeding, can make all the difference to how quickly she adapts to caring for the new member of the family. However, many people seem to expect mothers to be back to normal and doing everything they did before in a matter of days, which can make breastfeeding much more challenging than it should be.

Although the first couple of weeks are particularly crucial (which is why a babymoon is so valuable), most mothers continue to need help for several more weeks, while they adjust their lifestyle to accommodate their baby. But it needs to be the right sort of help.

How family and friends can help you

It can be hard for parents and other relatives who are used to formula feeding to understand why it's important for you to stay close to your baby and feed him whenever he asks. They may want to help by taking him away to settle him, so you can rest – or suggest that someone else give him a bottle feed occasionally, to give you a break. These offers of help are well-meant but they can seriously undermine breastfeeding.

'My mother-in-law told me she found a dummy a really useful way to keep her babies quiet if they woke up too early for a feed. I don't want to use a dummy but I didn't want to start an argument, so I just said "Really? Thanks – I'll remember that." She hasn't mentioned it again.'

Ashley, mother of Oliver, two weeks

Some mothers find the answer is to have a breastfeeding 'buddy' to encourage them and make it easier to turn down inappropriate offers of help, and to provide support through any breastfeeding problems. Your buddy could be your part-ner, your mother, a close friend, or even another breastfeeding mother you've only just met (see below).

One of the best ways friends and relatives can support you is to boost your confidence and respect your ability to choose what's right for your baby. While there will probably be times when you *do* want someone to look after him, mostly what you'll need is for others to make you snacks and drinks, and take over time-consuming tasks that keep you away from him.

Support from other mothers

There may be times when you need specific help with a breastfeeding problem, but there may also be times when you just want to meet other breastfeeding mothers, to exchange tips on everyday things, such as night-time feeds or dealing with teething. A breastfeeding support group or Baby Café™ can provide both types of help in an informal and friendly environment.

The availability of breastfeeding support groups varies enormously and you may find you need to travel some distance to get to one, especially if you live in a rural area. In the UK, most are run by volunteers with specialist training in breastfeeding. Some maternity departments, birthing centres and health centres run drop-in breastfeeding clinics that double up as support groups. Your midwife or health visitor should know what's available near you. Alternatively, you could contact the organisations listed in *Sources of information and support*, page 278, to find out whether they have a group in your area.

If you can't get to a group – or don't want to – you may be able to access the support or information you need by talking to someone on a breastfeeding helpline. These are run by trained breastfeeding supporters or counsellors who can help with specific problems, as well as providing a listening ear for mothers who are finding breastfeeding challenging and who simply want to 'offload'.

What to expect as your baby gets older

Breastfeeding changes and evolves as babies grow and mature. Mostly, these changes happen so gradually that you won't notice them until you look back, but it may be handy to know what to expect.

What to expect with your breasts

The amount of milk you make when you're breastfeeding is never static – your body responds to your baby's needs as they change. Once the setting-up period of the first few weeks is over, your breasts settle down to make what they're being asked to make, with just a bit to spare. Then, if they get a clear message that a different quantity is needed, they start to increase or decrease production.

The way your breasts feel will change as your baby grows. For the first few weeks they'll tend to feel full before a feed and softer afterwards. By about three months, as well as being less prone to leaking, they'll be noticeably softer most of the time. In fact, between feeds they'll probably feel like they did before you were pregnant.

This change shows that your breasts are now so in tune with your baby that they make milk extra-rapidly when he is feeding and more slowly at other times. It's *not* a sign that your milk is 'drying up'. If your three-month-old is happy and growing, soft breasts are a sign of how well breastfeeding is going.

Adapting as your baby gets bigger

As your baby grows, you'll need to start adjusting the way you hold him for feeding, to accommodate his longer legs and body. For example, if you have been used to cradling him at your breast, with your hand cupping his bottom, you may begin to find you can't reach that far – or that, if you do, his head is in the wrong position for feeding. You'll also need to work out a different way to support him, so you don't have all of his weight on your arm. If you don't allow for his changing size you may find that either your baby or your breast is getting squashed, which can lead to soreness, blocked ducts or mastitis for you, and frustration for him.

Many mothers instinctively solve the problem of holding a bigger baby by crossing their legs, so that they can support their baby's bottom on their thigh, allowing their hand to move up to his ribcage. The important thing is to experiment a bit and wriggle around until you find what works for you, rather than feeling you have to stick to a particular position. As he gets bigger still he'll become more agile and will be able to adapt his own position. (See page 168 for more on feeding older babies.)

If your baby gets distracted

As your baby gets older, he'll be increasingly interested in what's going on around him, which may mean he's easily distracted while he's feeding. He might pull away from the breast when he hears someone talking, or twist round (sometimes taking your nipple with him!) to look at the dog or the TV. This is fine if you've got plenty of time but if you need him to finish his feed quickly, it could be frustrating.

If you want your baby to concentrate on feeding, finding a quiet space to feed him, turning off the TV, making the room dark and talking soothingly or singing to him will all help. If you're out, draping a muslin or scarf over his head and face (or feeding him tucked up inside your T-shirt), will prevent other people's movements from catching his eye.

What happens when my baby is teething?

At some point during his first year your baby's teeth will begin to appear. The teeth themselves won't affect breastfeeding (because it's his tongue, not his gums, that squeezes out the milk), but he may decide to give your breast a little nip, especially if his gums are itchy.

If your baby does decide to bite you, it will usually happen at the end of a feed. Because his tongue covers his lower gum while he's feeding, he'll need to move it back so he doesn't bite that too, and he can't do this while he's feeding. (He is likely to know what will hurt *him* – but he won't understand what's likely to hurt *you*.) You'll soon learn to recognise when he's starting to do this, either by feeling his attachment alter or by detecting a change in his expression. This will allow you to gently remove him from your breast before he has a chance to bite.

'All of mine tried to bite me – but they only did it once or twice. I'm not sure whether that was because I learned to spot the gleam in their eye just before they did it, or because they were so stunned by the shriek I let out the first time that they didn't dare risk it again! Either way, it wasn't an issue for long.'

Bryony, mother of Patrick, 14 years, Freddie, 12 years,
and Amy, 10 years

If your baby goes on strike

Occasionally a baby will refuse to breastfeed for no apparent reason. If he's very young, the most likely explanation is that he is being held awkwardly (see page 42). But if he suddenly refuses to feed after a period of feeding with no problems, it may be that he is having a 'nursing strike'.

In a child of 18 months or older, a nursing strike may (or may not) mean that he is ready to stop breastfeeding for good. But this is very unlikely to be the case for a younger child, especially a baby under a year old, who is still reliant on milk. There are many things that can make a baby decide he doesn't want to be at the breast. For example:

- His mother's body tensed or jerked, or she gripped him suddenly while feeding. If he's teething maybe he bit her, which made her jump.
- An older child bit or smacked him while he was feeding.

- Someone close by shouted or made a sudden loud noise during a feed.
- Feeding hurts him, for example if he has an earache or is teething.
- The milk suddenly tastes unpleasant. This could be because his mother has eaten an unfamiliar, strongly flavoured food or it may be that she is starting a period, pregnant (see page 172) or developing mastitis (see page 240), all of which can change the taste of the breastmilk.
- He doesn't recognise his mother. (A radical change of hairstyle, an unusually croaky voice or an unfamiliar perfume can sometimes be enough to confuse a baby.)

If your baby has gone on strike, the first thing to do is work out why it's happening and, if you can, stop or avoid the cause. However, sometimes there's no obvious explanation or the trigger was a one-off event that appears to have had a lasting effect. In this case, the best option is to concentrate on helping your baby to rediscover your chest as a lovely, soothing place to be (see below). Feeding will probably follow naturally, once he realises that nothing horrible is going to happen.

OUCH – THAT HURTS!

Mothers are sometimes advised to breastfeed their baby while he is given an injection or has blood taken, to soothe him and take his mind off the pain. This is okay occasionally, but if your baby is having a series of injections or blood tests and discovers that every time he starts to feed he gets a sharp pain in his arm, leg or foot, he may decide that breastfeeding hurts and it's not worth the risk. It may be better to breastfeed after the jab rather than during it.

Helping your baby to get back to breastfeeding

The best way to help your baby overcome a suspicion of the breast is to tap into the instincts that were strongest for him when he was born. To help recreate that special time and make him feel safe:

- Make sure the room is nice and warm.
- Pull the curtains or dim the lights.
- Choose either complete quiet, soft music, 'white noise' or 'womb music'.
- Lie back and place your baby tummy-down on top of you, skin to skin. His head can be well away from your breasts – if he wants to feed, he'll wriggle into a feeding position by himself.
- He may cry at first; talk to him gently to help soothe him.
- Using a little warmed baby oil, massage his back, arms and legs with long, slow, downward strokes.
- Stay in this position as long as you can, even if he falls asleep. Babies often feed instinctively when they are just drifting off or waking up.
- Concentrate on rebuilding your relationship with your baby; feeding will follow.

Sharing a warm, relaxing bath may also help. Make sure the bathroom is warm and ask someone else to pass your baby to you once you're in the water. Lean back and lay him on your front, then pour water over him to keep him warm. A flannel over his back will help the warmth to spread evenly, so it doesn't startle him.

It's better if your baby is *not* desperately hungry when you try these ideas. If necessary, offer him a small feed of expressed breastmilk before you start, preferably in a beaker or a 'sippy' cup. Don't expect him to latch on and feed straight away. In fact, if he's been refusing the breast for a few days it may take more than one session before he feels confident enough to try. If he has been using a dummy you may want to stop this, at least temporarily, to encourage him to rediscover your breast as a source of comfort. Above all, don't rush him.

Key points

- Routines imposed by adults don't work for breast-feeding. Your baby's unique feeding pattern will emerge if you allow it to.

- Breastfeeding will get easier as you and your baby become more skilled, and your breasts settle down to match his needs.

- It's easy to breastfeed discretely if you need to when you're out and about.

- Friends and relatives can help you best by relieving you of other responsibilities, not by taking over the care of your baby.

- Other breastfeeding mothers can be a huge source of information and support, especially while you and your baby are settling in to breastfeeding.

- The way your baby feeds, and how you hold him for feeding, will evolve as breastfeeding progresses, and your breasts will feel less full most of the time.

- A period of breast refusal (or a 'nursing strike') doesn't necessarily mean the end of breastfeeding.

8

Lifestyle and breastfeeding

There are all sorts of myths about breastfeeding and issues such as diet, drinking, smoking, exercise and sex. Mostly, you don't need to make any changes to the things you enjoy in order to breastfeed but there are a few things that can have an impact, either on your general health or on how settled and healthy your baby is. This chapter aims to give you the facts about everyday lifestyle choices and breastfeeding.

What to eat when you're breastfeeding

Many people imagine that you need to eat a special diet, or avoid certain foods, in order to breastfeed. This isn't true.

TIP

Following your baby's lead with breastfeeding helps your body rhythms to match hers, so you may find you naturally want to eat and drink when she does. Make sure you have something handy to snack on whenever she feeds. If you make yourself a packed lunch first thing in the morning, you can grab it in the middle of the day. It's a good idea to keep a stock of nutritious 'fast foods', such as yoghurts, cheese, nuts and fruit in the house.

EATING FOR TWO?

You don't need to 'eat for two' when you're breastfeeding because your metabolism makes better use of what you're already eating. There's no need to make a point of drinking lots, either. Your body puts your baby first and adjusts your appetite to tell you how much you need to eat and drink to make up for what it uses to make milk. All you need do is to respond to what your body is telling you.

Whether or not you eat an ideal diet is very unlikely to have any effect on your breastmilk because your breasts take what your baby needs from your body stores. In countries throughout the world, women nourish their babies perfectly even though their own diets are poor – it's the mother's health that suffers first. However, giving birth and adjusting to life with a newborn are tiring. So, although you don't have to eat well to breastfeed, eating nothing but junk food will affect your energy levels and general wellbeing and may make looking after your baby harder.

It's not necessary to drink milk or eat meat to make nutritious breastmilk. However, mothers who eat a vegan or macrobiotic diet that contains *no* animal protein (in other words, no meat, fish, eggs or dairy foods) should take supplements of vitamin B12, to be sure that they and their baby get enough of this important vitamin.

There aren't any foods that should be avoided by every breastfeeding mother. In fact, most babies actively enjoy strong flavours, such as garlic, in breastmilk. The only foods you shouldn't eat are those that you may have been advised to avoid because of severe allergies in the family (although so far there is no clear evidence to show that this will definitely help to prevent your baby developing allergies later).

Mothers sometimes wonder, if their baby is unusually unsettled for a few hours, whether the cause might be something they ate. For example, cabbage and baked beans are often blamed for giving babies wind. But it's the roughage in these foods that causes wind – and roughage can't get into your bloodstream, or your milk. Fizzy drinks can sometimes make babies irritable but it's the caffeine in them that's to blame (see below), not the bubbles. If you think something you've eaten may have upset your baby, test it by eating it once or twice more (with a few days' gap in between) before you decide to cut it from your diet.

Caffeine passes into breastmilk and because it's a stimulant, it can sometimes make babies irritable. It doesn't get into the milk in great quantities but it stays in a baby's system longer than it does in an adult's, so the levels can build up. While the odd fizzy drink or cup of coffee may give *you* a quick 'buzz', having too many could end up making your baby unsettled over a longer period. Generally, anything under five cups of coffee a day is probably okay, but every baby is different. If your baby seems miserable for no apparent reason, try cutting down your caffeine intake for a week or so to see if it helps.

Very occasionally, a baby who is constantly miserable or has a persistent rash seems to get better if her mother stops eating a particular food (for example, dairy foods). If you suspect your baby may be reacting to a fundamental part of your diet, it's best to consult a doctor or dietitian before making big changes.

Do I need extra vitamin D?

The production of vitamin D is triggered by sunlight and exposing our skin to a reasonable amount of sun should normally allow us to make what we need. However, the lack of strong sunlight throughout the year in the UK means that many adults and children are at risk of vitamin D deficiency.

Because of this, all women who are pregnant or breastfeeding are advised to take a vitamin D supplement and routine supplements of vitamin D, together with vitamins A and C, are recommended for babies after they reach six months. (Infant formula has the supplement already added.)

Some people are at particular risk of vitamin D deficiency. They include those who:

- have dark skin
- wear clothing that prevents their skin being exposed to sunlight
- routinely cover any exposed skin with high-factor sun creams
- rarely go outside the house
- have a body mass index (BMI) of 30 or over.

Babies whose mothers fall into one of these categories may be born with low levels of vitamin D and the amount in breast-milk is unlikely to be enough for them on its own. The risk is higher still if the baby has dark skin or is rarely exposed to the sun. The current recommendation is that these babies, if they are breastfed, should be given a vitamin D supplement from birth. Ask your midwife for advice.

Can I drink alcohol?

Small amounts are okay, but alcohol can interfere with the let-down reflex, so your baby may get slightly less milk than usual while it's in your system. But, provided you don't drink frequently, she will easily make up for this at her next few feeds. Alcohol also passes into breastmilk, so it will have similar effects on your baby to those it has on you. However, her liver is immature and less able than yours to deal with it, so while the occasional single drink is unlikely to cause her any harm, anything more than this could be risky.

Although alcohol gets into breastmilk it also leaves it, with time. This is useful to know, especially if you want to have more than the occasional single drink. The level of alcohol in your milk rises at the same rate as the level in your bloodstream (peaking around 30 to 60 minutes later) and subsides as your blood level goes down, taking about three hours for a single unit of alcohol to be completely out of your system.

If you want to have a drink but are keen to minimise the effect on your baby, here's what to do:

- Offer your baby a feed immediately *before* you have your drink.
- Have something to eat with your drink to help keep your blood alcohol level low.
- Try not to feed your baby for at least two hours after you've finished your drink.

There's no need to express your milk and throw it away (or 'pump and dump') to get rid of the alcohol; your body will deal with it naturally, in its own time.

The more you drink, the more time the alcohol will take to leave your system. **If you're planning an evening with several drinks it's a good idea to express some milk during the day, so that you (or someone else) can give this expressed milk to your baby later.** You will probably find you need to express some milk during the evening, too, in order to stay comfortable, but this is for *your* benefit, not your baby's. It won't affect the amount of alcohol she gets at her next feed – only time will do that.

'Lots of my friends who've had babies don't breastfeed because they think they won't be able to drink or go out. But I didn't want to go out all the time anyway after I had Lucia. And when I did I'd express some milk and my sister would feed her. It wasn't a big deal. Now my friends have seen the comfort she gets from the breast and how easy it is, they say they'd think about it next time.'

Irene, mother of Lucia, 11 months

Taking over-the-counter medicines

Most medicines are safe to take while breastfeeding and an alternative is usually available for the few that aren't. The majority either don't get into breastmilk or do so only in extremely small amounts. However, this isn't always clear. The leaflet that accompanies a medicine often states that it should not be taken while breastfeeding even though it can be quite safe to do so. This is because testing a drug for safety during lactation isn't required legally and costs time and money, so it often doesn't get done.

Over-the-counter medicines such as paracetamol, ibuprofen, antacids and haemorrhoid treatments can all be taken at normal dosages without presenting a risk to your baby. Most asthma medication and the current flu vaccine are safe. However, there are some medicines to avoid:

- Decongestants (such as pseudoephedrine) can drastically reduce milk production.
- Codeine can make babies sleepy.
- Aspirin is not safe for babies and young children.
- Some hay fever remedies can make babies drowsy (eye drops and nasal sprays don't get absorbed into the bloodstream, so they are safe to use).

Some herbal remedies can also present a risk to either the baby or the milk supply and, since they are not regulated and controlled, the strength of even 'safe' products is very variable. If in doubt, ask the in-store pharmacist for advice.

There has been little research into the possible effects of dental work on breastmilk, but it's thought the amount of mercury in a single filling would be too small to do any harm. The anaesthetic used in routine dental work is safe, although adrenaline is sometimes added to minimise bleeding and this can occasionally make a very sensitive baby irritable. Tell your dentist you are breastfeeding before planning any treatment.

The Breastfeeding Network (BfN) has online information about the safety of drugs for breastfeeding mothers, with a helpline for more unusual queries (see *Sources of information and support*, page 278).

Can I go on a diet?

Almost all mothers put on weight while they are pregnant. Some of this extra weight goes into making breastmilk, so in theory your pregnancy weight should disappear gradually and consistently over the first few months. However, not all women find that this works in practice and many want to speed up the process. It used to be said that breastfeeding mothers shouldn't try to lose weight but current evidence suggests that avoiding excess calories causes no problems for either mother or baby. Sudden 'crash dieting' or eating anything less than 1,800 calories per day is not a good idea, though.

Is it okay to exercise?

Moderate exercise is a good thing for a breastfeeding mother. It helps you to stay fit, gets your shape back after pregnancy and relieves stress. In the past, it was thought that extreme exercise might make babies refuse to breastfeed because of high levels of lactic acid in their mothers' breastmilk (which could make the milk taste odd) but research suggests this isn't a problem. In general, if exercising feels good, it's probably fine for both of you. But if it makes you very tired or dehydrated, it might be a good idea to scale it down.

What if I smoke?

If you can't manage to give up smoking, it's *much* better for your baby to be breastfed than to have formula. Breastfeeding helps to prevent illnesses such as bronchitis, pneumonia and ear infections, which are otherwise more common in babies whose mothers smoke. **The biggest risk is from the smoke itself, not from the ingredients of smoke that make it into your milk,** so the most important thing is to avoid smoking near your baby, or in the rooms in which she spends a lot of time.

Breastfeeding has been shown to lower the risk of sudden infant death syndrome (cot death), but sharing a bed with a smoker is known to *increase* the risk – even if no one smokes in the bedroom. So while keeping your baby near you at night is still recommended if you or your partner smoke, having her in your bed isn't. (See page 114 for more on safe bed sharing.)

Although the main risk to your baby's health is from breathing smoke, nicotine is not particularly good for her either – and the concentration of nicotine in your milk is three times higher than it is in your blood. The best way to reduce the amount of nicotine your baby gets is to smoke immediately *after* a breastfeed – or, if you're gasping for a cigarette, to offer her a quick feed before you light up.

CANNABIS IS NOT AN OPTION

The active ingredient in cannabis (marijuana) accumulates in breast-milk, with the level rising to as much as eight times that in the mother's bloodstream. It is also stored in body fat, meaning it can stay in a mother's system (and in her milk) for several weeks after she last smoked (or ate) it. At the very least it can make a baby sleepy and reluctant to feed but the long-term effects may be much more serious. You should avoid cannabis (and other street drugs) while you are breastfeeding.

Nicotine patches are safe to use while breastfeeding. However, patches deliver a steady level of nicotine throughout the day, so the level in your milk will be constant. Use the lowest-strength patches you can to replace the amount of nicotine your body is used to. If you opt for lozenges or gum, fit them around your baby's feeds as described above, to minimise the amount of nicotine she gets.

Your sex life

Caring for a baby can be exhausting. While some mothers say breastfeeding makes them feel extra sexy, it's not unusual for a couple's sex life to take a dive when they first become parents. But it's not just tiredness. Breastfeeding, cuddling and carrying involve a lot of physical contact, so at the end of a full-on day of mothering, it can be hard to share your body yet again. Simply having an hour or so to relax while someone else looks after the baby may help.

When you do manage a bit of intimacy, you may need to adapt what you do to accommodate the fact that you are breastfeeding. While positions that were uncomfortable during pregnancy will now be possible again, it's likely your breasts may feel more tender than before you were pregnant, especially when they're full. In general, sex will probably be more enjoyable and comfortable if you time it for just after a feed. Be ready for the 'love' hormone to trigger your let-down reflex as things hot up (see page 25) and perhaps warn your partner that you may leak milk.

Using breastfeeding as a contraceptive

Breastfeeding naturally prevents a quick return to fertility, to allow the mother's body to concentrate on nourishing the baby she is feeding rather than on growing a new one. As

The Lactational Amenorrhoea Method of contraception (LAM)

Breastfeeding can be as reliable as other commonly used methods of contraception, provided that:

- The baby is under six months old.
- The mother hasn't had a period since her baby was born.
- The baby is having only breastmilk, with no other foods or drinks (including water).
- The baby is feeding frequently, during the day and at night, with no more than one gap of longer than four hours (but not longer than six) in every 24.

long as the baby feeds frequently and has no other food or drink, the level of prolactin in the mother's bloodstream will stay high enough to override her normal menstrual cycle, preventing her from ovulating. This means that breastfeeding *can* be a reliable contraceptive, but only if certain rules are followed (see box, above).

If you are breastfeeding frequently and exclusively you're unlikely to have a period for at least six months after your baby is born – and possibly quite a bit longer. Some women are alerted to their first post-birth period by their baby temporarily rejecting the breast, because hormonal changes make their breastmilk taste slightly different. However, this is not a reliable way of telling whether or not you are fertile again, since it's possible you'll ovulate for the first time *before* you have your first period. If you don't want to rely on breastfeeding to prevent you becoming pregnant again, or if your baby is older than six months, it's advisable to use another method too.

Most contraceptive methods that involve hormones, such as the combined pill or injections, can reduce breastmilk production, although some mothers find they can start taking the mini pill after the first six weeks without a problem. However, synthetic hormones can also be passed to the baby through breastmilk and many mothers prefer to avoid the pill for this reason. For most breastfeeding couples, a barrier method of contraception, such as a cap (diaphragm) or condoms, is a better bet. Non-hormonal types of intrauterine device (contraceptive coil) may be suitable, too. If you go to a doctor or family planning nurse for contraceptive advice, be sure to let them know you're breastfeeding.

Key points

- A mother's body looks after her baby first so you don't need to have a perfect diet to breastfeed. But if your diet is poor you may find caring for your baby more tiring.

- There's no need to avoid particular foods while you're breastfeeding unless you have been advised to because of allergies.

- Occasionally something in a mother's diet may make her baby unsettled. Caffeine is a common culprit.

- Babies in certain high-risk groups may need to be given vitamin D supplements from birth.

- The occasional glass of alcohol is okay but anything more may affect your baby.

- Most over-the-counter medicines are safe to take while breastfeeding; if in doubt, check with a pharmacist or online.

- Dieting is safe while you're breastfeeding as long as it isn't too extreme or sudden.

- It's safe to exercise when you're breastfeeding as long as you don't overdo it.

- If you smoke, your baby is likely to be healthier if you breastfeed her than if you don't. Try to minimise the amount of smoke she breathes – and don't share a bed with her.

- Your breasts may be more tender during sex than they were before pregnancy, and you may leak milk.

- Breastfeeding can be a reliable contraceptive for the first six months, as long as you follow certain rules.

9

When you can't be with your baby

If there are times when you need to leave your baby with someone else, whether it's the odd evening out at the cinema or going back to work or study full time, breastfeeding can continue to be baby-led. There's no need to introduce bottles or get your baby into a routine for the times when you are apart. Understanding how your milk production works is key: you can be led by your baby when you are with him and, for the most part, by how your breasts feel when you aren't. Frequent feeding when you're together can help to make up for the time you have to spend apart, both physically (in terms of milk production) and emotionally, in terms of your relationship.

This chapter is about how to manage different kinds of separations so you can continue to meet your baby's needs. (The issues will be slightly different if you and your baby are separated because one of you is ill – see Chapter 14 – or if your baby is born early and is in a neonatal unit – see Chapter 11.)

How can I provide milk for my baby while we are apart?

If you are apart from your baby for more than a couple of hours while he's fully breastfed (i.e. younger than around six months), you'll need to leave him some milk. The younger he is, the more he'll need. The best milk for your baby is your breastmilk. Milk that has been expressed within the previous 24 hours is ideal, because it contains active, up-to-date anti-bodies, but milk that has been refrigerated for three to eight days (see table on page 151) is a good alternative. Breastmilk will also keep for up to six months in a freezer (see page 150), so you can build up a reserve stock in advance, if necessary. This will give you something to fall back on occasionally if you don't have enough freshly expressed.

An alternative to giving your baby your own milk is for another breastfeeding mother to breastfeed him when you can't be there. Before the days of formula milks, co-feeding (or 'wet nursing', as it used to be called), was widely prac-tised, and there are lots of mothers who are very happy to share breastfeeding with, say, a sister or close friend. Although each mother's milk is specifically made for her own baby, the differences between one mother's milk and the next are very small and some people find this preferable to using formula. If you're considering this, it's best to check beforehand that you and your friend agree about issues such as alcohol, caffeine and medicines, which your baby could be exposed to in the milk he receives – and to make sure both your partners are happy with the arrangement.

'I shared breastfeeding with a friend. I never really thought about it when I was pregnant but it made so much sense. I'd look after her baby now and then and feed him if he was hungry – and she'd feed Caitlin if I went out. I never managed to express much milk, so sharing breastfeeding meant neither of us had to bother with bottles or formula.'

Julie, mother of Caitlin, three years, and Freddie, 11 months

The third option is for your baby to have formula when you can't be with him. This avoids you having to express milk in advance but it disturbs some of the protective effects for his

> ### TIP
>
> If your baby is older than about eight months, and has started eating some solid foods, he may be able to go for several hours without a milk feed – as long as he's able to feed frequently enough to make up for it (especially during the night) when you are together again.

health of having only breastmilk (and it can be expensive). However, many mothers find that, for regular separations, this is a workable choice that allows them to keep breast-feeding going. See page 153 for information on combining formula with breastfeeding.

The following few sections deal with expressing so that your baby can have your milk while you are separated. Even if you choose co-feeding or to give him formula, you will need to express at least some breastmilk while you are apart, to prevent overfullness and maintain your milk production. You can be led by how your breasts feel. Just express enough to keep yourself comfortable – and feed your baby again as soon as you can. If the separation is longer, or repeated regularly (for example if you are going back to work or college), expressing at roughly the times when he would usually be feeding will keep your breasts producing milk at a steady rate. **If you have to leave your baby in the first two weeks, you'll need to express frequently while you're apart, so that the setting-up of your capacity for long-term milk production isn't affected.**

Putting in an advance order for expressed milk

Breastfeeding works on the principle of production according to demand. So, by the time he's a few weeks old, you'll be producing as much milk as your baby needs – but not a lot more. This means that if you try to express you may not get much at all, especially immediately after a breastfeed. Expressing and freezing small amounts now and then is a useful way to build up a small store in case you need it unexpectedly, but if you want your breasts to come up with extra milk on a regular basis, you'll have to give them a bit of notice. It's all about putting in the order.

What if I have to leave my baby for an afternoon?

If you're going to be away from your baby for only a few hours, and you have a day or two's notice, you should be able to get away with expressing three or four times during that period, and storing the milk in the fridge (see page 150). If you haven't previously been expressing regularly you may not be able to express enough for a really satisfying feed but – unless your baby is very young – this won't matter. Provided he has something to take the edge off his hunger, he'll make up for it when you're back together.

How can I prepare to go back to work?

If you're going back to work or college, it's a good idea to have a reasonable store of expressed milk in your freezer as a 'buffer' while you are getting to grips with the changes. This

TIP

If you leak milk from one breast while feeding from the other, you can collect this 'drip milk' in a drip catcher (see page 79) and freeze it. However, milk that leaks freely at the beginning of a breastfeed tends to be low in fat, so a feed consisting entirely of drip milk may not satisfy your baby's hunger for long. It's fine for the occasional short-term separation but is unlikely to be sufficient on its own for long-term use.

will also give you peace of mind if you go through a temporary downward 'blip' in milk production, which can happen if you are exceptionally busy. It's best to start building up your store *at least* a few days before you're going to need to start using expressed milk, and preferably a few weeks.

To express and save milk in advance, you need to put in an order for more than your baby currently needs. The best way to do this is to mimic the way he asks for extra feeds during an 'appetite spurt', when he needs to increase your supply. This means expressing milk regularly between feeds (especially in any longer gaps), and expressing from the second breast whenever your baby feeds only (or mainly) from one. (Expressing just after your baby has fed can also work, although you'll probably get less out at first that way.)

Your baby is likely to be far more efficient at getting milk out of your breasts than either your hands or a breast pump, so don't worry if the amounts you express are small, especially at first. Breastfed babies rarely take as much milk during a feed (or even during a whole day) as babies on formula, so your baby won't need or expect huge quantities. Fitting in two or three expressing sessions over 24 hours means your breasts will quickly get the message and start to make more. You'll probably notice a difference within a day or two: they'll feel slightly fuller and you'll be getting more milk each time. The secret, though, is to focus on putting in the order, rather than on the quantities you're getting out.

Once you go back to work or college you should aim to express roughly as many times as your baby would have fed (or more often). In practice, however, most mothers who work full time don't manage to express more than about three times a day and many get by with fewer. (See page 157 for information on expressing at work.) The key is to listen to your body and express as soon as your breasts start to feel full – and to encourage your baby to breastfeed as much as possible when you are not at work, to make up for any missed sessions.

'By about ten months the amounts I expressed were getting smaller and smaller, probably because Poppy was probably drinking less during the day. I stopped expressing but carried on breastfeeding in the morning, evening and night. She'd usually have a long feed before I went to work and she'd be on the breast lots when I was home. She just had solids during the day.'

Alison, mother of Jack, four years, and Poppy, two years

What happens if I need to leave my baby for more than a day?

Occasionally, mothers need to provide milk for their baby for a day or two, with only a few days' notice, perhaps because of work or social commitments or because they need to stop breastfeeding temporarily for a medical reason. If you want your baby to continue to have only your milk but you don't have a stock to fall back on you'll need to express intensively in any available time to stockpile as much as you can.

To increase your milk production rapidly, set yourself a target of expressing as often as you possibly can, both after feeds and between feeds, draining your breasts as fully as possible each time (see *How to give your breasts a two-week 'wake-up call'*, page 189, for tips on maximising the amount you express). Provided you don't express immediately before your baby is likely to want a big feed, you will still have enough milk for him. (If he wants to feed more often because there isn't quite as much there as usual, that will help to stimulate your breasts even more.) Focus on putting in the order, not on what you're getting out each time.

If the separation happens immediately after this period of intense expressing, you'll probably need to express frequently to stay comfortable (and prevent engorgement) while you and your baby are apart, because of the increased production you've generated. However, if you're not aiming to save the milk (perhaps because it contains a drug that your baby mustn't have), there's no need to wash and sterilise any equipment you use.

Once you and your baby are back together it will take a little while for your needs and his to get back in sync, so don't be surprised if his usual feeding pattern takes a day or two to return.

'I went on a two-day business trip when Lola was 15 months. I took the pump with me and expressed in the hotel room to keep comfortable. I was surprised how full I got, even so – she was obviously still drinking a lot of milk, even though she wasn't having it during the day. By the time I got home the next evening my boobs felt like they were exploding. I had to wake her up to feed. She was so happy – she said "Mummy!", then "Booby!"'

Sam, mother of Lola, two years

How to express your milk

You can express your milk by hand or with a pump – or you can use a combination of both methods. Hand expression (see page 86) has several advantages over pumping and, with a bit of practice, it can be just as quick. If you practise expressing by hand first, you'll be able to decide whether or not you need a pump as well. You'll need to wash your hands before expressing milk to be given to your baby.

When you feed your baby, your let-down reflex operates without you having to think about it but when you express your milk you may find it needs a little help, especially if you're using a pump. One solution is to express from one breast while feeding your baby from the other. This works particularly well if you're very full and he is likely to want only one breast, but it can be a bit fiddly to manage, especially if he's inclined to wriggle. If you want to express when he's not feeding, cuddling him skin to skin can be a good way to trigger the let-down reflex.

If you need to express and haven't got your baby near you, you can stimulate your let-down reflex in other ways. Each woman's oxytocin triggers are different, so feel free to experiment to find what works for you. Remember that oxytocin is the 'love hormone'; it can easily be turned off if you don't feel relaxed, comfortable and safe, so take some time to focus and get in the mood, if you need to. The box below contains some ideas that may help (although the ones you can use in a work environment might be limited!)

There's no need to watch the clock when you're expressing; your milk flow is a much more useful guide as to how long you should keep going. If you're trying to get as much milk as possible, keep expressing as long as you're getting milk then switch to the other breast. When the flow subsides on that one, switch back to the first. This will trigger a new let-down and release another rush of milk.

Ideas for encouraging your let-down reflex

- a photo or video of your baby
- an item of your baby's clothing (worn, so it smells of him)
- a recording of your baby squeaking or murmuring
- a warm bath, or warm flannels laid over your breasts
- a warm drink
- relaxing music
- low lighting
- relaxation techniques – perhaps some you practised for use in labour
- gentle breast massage or stimulation – whatever feels nice but nothing too deep. The purpose isn't to push milk down the ducts but to get your oxytocin going
- if you like, your partner can cuddle you, talk soothingly to you, give you a back massage, or touch and stroke your breasts.

Expressing from both breasts at once can be very effective at triggering the let-down reflex and stimulating milk production, as well as cutting down the time you need to spend. Some electric pumps are equipped for double pumping; if you're expressing by hand you'll find it easier to catch the milk, and less messy, if you use a really wide bowl or jug.

There's no advantage in continuing to express if nothing much is coming out. Switching to the other breast, doing some gentle breast massage or nipple stimulation, or simply taking a break (even for a couple of minutes) will do more to stimulate both milk flow and milk production than slogging away at it when nothing is happening.

How do I choose a breast pump?

There are lots of different breast pumps on the market. If possible, talk to friends who have used a pump – perhaps even try theirs – and look on the Internet, before deciding which type will suit you best. The more time you will be spending apart from your baby and the more keen you are to ensure he has only your milk, the more likely you are to need a sophisticated pump – but size and portability will be important too.

Hand-operated pumps have either a bulb or a handle, which you squeeze to create a vacuum. The degree of suction is controlled by how hard and how long you squeeze. Electric pumps run on battery or mains power, or both, with a dial for setting your preferred strength. **Although some are quieter than others, all electric pumps make a noise when they're working – worth bearing in mind if you want to be able to use your pump at work discreetly!** All pumps come apart for cleaning and sterilising, though some are trickier than others to re-assemble.

If you need to pump intensively, short term – for example, if your baby is in hospital (see page 250) – you can hire an electric pump from organisations such as the NCT (see

Sources of information and support, page 278). However, if you are going back to work, it's probably cheaper and more convenient to buy your own.

The size of the funnel can make a difference to how much milk you get. If the pump you choose comes with more than one funnel it's worth experimenting to see if one works better than the other. It's also important to start expressing gently and build up the suction gradually until you find the intensity that's best for you. Strong suction isn't necessarily good or effective, so there's no need to feel you have to get to the maximum setting.

How to store breastmilk

The recommendations in this section refer to milk that is being stored for a healthy baby to drink in a home environment or day nursery. See Chapter 11 for what to do if your baby is in a neonatal unit.

Breastmilk can be stored in a feeding bottle, a specially designed sterile bag, or a food-safe plastic container that has been thoroughly cleaned and then scalded with boiling water. Unlike made-up formula, it doesn't go off easily because it contains living cells that stop bacteria multiplying, so it can safely be stored for quite long periods.

At normal room temperature, breastmilk will be safe for six hours – and it can be kept for about eight hours in a cool bag with ice packs. (Make sure the ice packs don't touch the milk container, so the milk doesn't freeze.) **There's no need to refrigerate milk you express to be given to your baby within a few hours.**

Breastmilk will keep for about a week in a fridge that is at a constant temperature of less than 4°C. However, most domestic fridges aren't kept that low. Three days is fine as long as the temperature doesn't rise above 10°C. Keep the milk at the back of the fridge rather than in the door, to be sure.

Breastmilk can be stored in a freezer (at a temperature of –18°C or lower) for up to six months. Saving it in small amounts will make it easier and less wasteful to defrost. Each new batch should be frozen separately rather than added to a container that already has frozen milk in it. Label each one with the date of expressing.

Frozen breastmilk is best defrosted slowly, in a fridge, and used within 12 hours. If you need it more quickly than this, defrost it by standing the container in hand-hot water and shaking it gently every few minutes. Fully defrosted breastmilk should be used immediately. Freezing and defrosting can cause milk to separate but that doesn't mean it's not safe to use; a quick, gentle shake is all that's needed to mix the cream back in. However, if the milk smells sour, throw it away – and don't refreeze milk that's been frozen and defrosted.

There's no need to heat breastmilk before offering it to your baby – and *over*heating it may destroy some of the protective antibodies. However, many babies don't like milk straight from the fridge, in which case taking it out half an hour before you need it, or warming it slightly by standing the bottle or beaker in a jug of hand-hot water for a minute or two, is all that's needed. **Never heat breastmilk in a microwave oven or a saucepan – you risk overheating it and destroying some of its valuable ingredients, as well as possibly scalding your baby's mouth.**

Quick guide to storing breastmilk

Where/what temperature	Milk will keep up to:
Room temperature	6 hours
Cool bag with ice packs	8 hours
Fridge (maximum temp. 10°C)	3 days
Fridge (maximum temp. 4°C)	8 days
Freezer (maximum temp. −18°C)	6 months

Should I introduce a bottle?

Breastfeeding mothers are sometimes advised to get their baby used to a bottle as early as possible so that he will accept one later. However, introducing a bottle when your baby is still learning to breastfeed can cause problems. Feeding from a teat is different from breastfeeding (see page 34) and he may find it difficult to switch between one and the other if he is asked to learn both at the same time. (Contrary to what some adverts say, there is no teat on sale that is really 'like a breast', because your breast moulds itself to the shape of your baby's mouth when he feeds, and changes shape as he sucks and swallows.) For short separations, it may be better to feed a very young baby with a small cup (see box, below).

If you do decide to use a bottle while your baby is still very young, try to ensure that whoever is feeding him coaxes him to use the same sort of technique he needs to use for breastfeeding, rather than poking the teat into his mouth. Touching the teat against his nose will encourage him to open his mouth wide and stick his tongue out, so that he 'scoops' it up. This will help him to remember what to do when he's breastfeeding.

Babies who are efficient at breastfeeding can generally work out how to use a teat, and will switch back to the breast without difficulty. And babies older than six months (some as

How to feed a young baby using a cup

Cup feeding is a useful way to give small amounts of milk to a baby who is still learning to breastfeed, so that he can avoid using a bottle. The cup needs to be small, to reduce the risk of accidental choking. A shot glass, medicine measure, egg cup or the cover from a feeding bottle are all about the right size. Check that the rim is smooth and rounded and not too thick. Wash the cup in hot, soapy water and rinse it well.

To cup feed a baby:

- Fill the cup about three-quarters full to start with, so it won't spill easily but won't need to be tipped too much either.
- Wrap the baby so that his arms can't knock the cup.
- Sit him upright on your lap, with the heel of your hand on his upper back.
- Support his neck with the fingers and thumb of the same hand, so that he can lift his chin slightly.
- Rest the cup gently on the baby's lower lip and tilt it so that the milk touches his upper lip.
- Wait for him to start lapping or sipping. *Don't be tempted to pour milk into his mouth, because that could make him choke.*
- Leave the cup in place, adjusting the tilt to keep the milk touching the baby's top lip.
- Let him take the milk at his own pace. It's important that the baby is in control of the feed. (Be prepared for him trying to suck, which may be messy.)
- Be ready to top up the cup with more milk when it gets down to about a quarter full.

young as four months) are usually able to manage a beaker or a 'sippy cup' by themselves, in which case there's no need to introduce a bottle at all.

Bottles and teats need to be thoroughly cleaned and then sterilised, either by boiling for 10 minutes, immersing in a cold water sterilising solution for at least 30 minutes, or putting through the programme of a steam steriliser. Cups (especially open cups with no lid or spout) are easier than bottles to clean and dry thoroughly, so the risk of germs breeding in them is less. Unless your baby is premature or at particular risk of infection, a cup just needs to be thoroughly cleaned in hot soapy water and rinsed well.

What if I decide to use formula?

If you decide that your baby will have formula feeds when you can't be with him there are a few things it may be useful to know about which formula to choose and how to prepare the feeds.

An infant (stage 1) formula is the best substitute for breastmilk. 'Hungrier baby milks' and 'follow-on milks' are not necessary (and tend to be more expensive). Most brands of formula come in ready-made and powdered forms. Ready-made feeds are convenient, and their sterility is guaranteed but they, too, tend to be expensive. Powdered formula is generally cheaper but it is not necessarily sterile, even when the box or tin has only just been opened. **Adding water to the powder allows any bacteria in the milk to start reproducing, so powdered formula feeds should be made up freshly each time, not prepared in advance.** Make sure your baby's carer knows how to make up a formula feed (see box, below).

If your baby has followed a typical breastfeeding pattern you may find that he prefers to stick to small, frequent feeds and that he needs less formula at each feed than the instructions

How to make up a formula feed

If your baby is going to be feeding from a small cup, or a beaker or 'sippy' cup with no quantity markings on the side, it will need to be made up in a sterilised feeding bottle and then transferred to the cup. (A small measuring jug will do but the feed will need to be stirred thoroughly to mix it.)

To make up a formula feed:

- Use recently boiled tap water (not bottled water, which can be high in salt), at about 70°C.
- Measure the right amount of water into the bottle.
- Using the scoop provided, add the correct amount of powder, levelling off the scoop with a flat edge (such as the back of a knife blade).
- Shake well to mix the feed.
- Cool to a safe temperature, preferably under running cold water.
- Throw away any unused milk.

on the packet suggest. It's important to explain this to whoever is looking after him. If he has not previously been given feeds by bottle, persuading him to accept one may take gentleness and perseverance (see below). If he is older than four or five months he may prefer a beaker or 'sippy cup' to a bottle.

What if my baby refuses to be fed?

Some babies won't accept feeds from a bottle or a cup and this can make separations stressful for everyone concerned. Partners and grandparents can feel hurt and anxious if they can't persuade the baby to feed, while knowing your baby won't take milk from anyone else may make leaving him extra difficult for you. Offering a feed before the baby is truly hungry can sometimes help but trying to force a baby to take a feed when he is clearly saying no is likely to lead to more problems, not fewer.

> 'I went back to work when Ava was six months and I was really worried because she refused to have a bottle or a cup. I thought she'd starve. Right up until the day I started work I didn't know what would happen. But on the first day our nanny gave her a bottle and just let her play with it. She eventually worked out how to do it herself. The nanny wasn't worried – she knew Ava would work out what to do as she'd done it with lots of other babies. So she was fine from the first day.'
>
> *Tania, mother of Ava, 18 months*

Babies don't starve themselves. Your baby will be okay, even if he ends up waiting until you get back at the end of the day before he has a feed. Many breastfeeding babies whose mothers are at work or college decide to manage without milk while Mummy isn't there – and make up for it by feeding frequently when she is. And many breastfeeding mothers are more than happy to spend time catching up on their relationship with their baby when they are back together.

If your baby decides to go on feeding strike during the day and make up for lost time at night, you will probably want to make sure feeding at night is as easy as possible for both of you – see page 113 for some tips. You may need to be prepared to allow extra time in the mornings for your baby to have a good feed before you leave him, and to spend most of the evening with him at your breast.

Whether or not your baby is happy to be fed by someone else, being fed with a bottle or cup won't feel the same to him as breastfeeding so it's important that whoever is feeding him holds him close during the feed and gives him plenty of cuddles.

How do I manage going back to work?

When your baby is newborn, the thought of organising your life to allow you to go back to work can be daunting enough without thinking about how you will manage breastfeeding. However, by the time you go back your baby will be older. He'll have established his feeding pattern and feeds won't take as long. If you're not returning to work until six months or more after the birth, he may well be having some solid foods as well, so he won't be totally reliant on breastmilk. This will make it easier for others to share his feeding.

'I'm really glad I was still breastfeeding when I went back to work. The separation would have been much harder if I'd stopped breastfeeding at the same time. Because I was still feeding her we could bond again in the evening and at night-time – that was really important for both of us.'

Beth, mother of Martha, 15 months

If commuting with your baby is a practical option, choosing a nursery or childminder near to your work or college, rather than your home, will shorten the time you have to spend away from him. This can mean you don't have to miss as many feeds, and you may even be able to breastfeed during your lunch break.

If you want to feed your baby at lunchtimes and/or when you pick him up, make sure his carer knows when you will arrive and ask them to make sure they don't give him a feed just before you get there. If your baby is being cared for by a relative, nanny or childminder (rather than in a nursery), ask if they can bring him to your workplace at lunchtime so you can feed him there.

It's easy when bottle feeding (or spoon feeding) to persuade a baby to take more than he needs, which can disrupt his usual breastfeeding pattern. If possible, explain to your baby's carer that he is used to deciding how much he needs and that small feeds (or just a little solid food) are fine by you. It may be worth explaining that formula-fed babies almost always require more milk than breastfed babies because formula contains ingredients that can't be fully digested.

It's a good idea to have a few days' trial run with your childcare arrangements before you return to work or college, so you can iron out any issues in advance. This will help you to feel more relaxed and confident on your first day back.

Tips for expressing at work

Expressing milk for your baby while you are at work takes a bit of forward planning. Many mothers find they have more milk at the beginning of their working week than towards the end, so they focus on expressing milk most intensively in the first few days. Having something with you that reminds you of your baby will help you to get your let-down reflex to work (see *Ideas for encouraging your let-down reflex*, page 147). And you may find it useful to keep a supply of 'wet wipes', breast pads and a spare top and bra at work, in case of leaks.

Employers are bound by health and safety legislation to do what they can to enable mothers to keep breastfeeding. Once you have told your employer (in writing) that you will be breastfeeding when you return to work, they will have to carry out a risk assessment to ensure that your working conditions don't present a danger to you or your baby (for example, through contamination of your breastmilk). You can also ask to have your hours adjusted to make life easier – for example, a longer lunch break, to allow you to visit your baby to feed him, or a shorter break or earlier start, to enable you to get away earlier at the end of the day.

Your employer must also allow you 'rest' breaks, which you can use for feeding or expressing, and you must be provided with privacy and a clean and safe place for you to express and store your milk. You may be able to negotiate the use of a fridge, although a cool bag with ice packs will do

TELL YOUR EMPLOYER!

Supporting you to continue breastfeeding is in your employer's interests. Breastfeeding means your baby will continue to receive his daily update of live antibodies (see page 7), which will reduce the chances of him becoming ill and requiring you to take time off work to look after him. Breastfeeding also boosts *your* immunity and helps to regulate your metabolism, so you are less likely to be ill.

instead (see page 149). See *Sources of information and support*, page 278, for details of organisations that can provide further information on your rights as a breastfeeding working mother.

Key points

- You can keep breastfeeding going, even if you can't be with your baby all the time.

- If you have to be apart from your baby you can express and store your milk for him. Alternatively, someone else can breastfeed him or you can introduce some formula.

- You can express your milk by hand or with a pump – or use a combination of both.

- When you first start expressing you may not get much milk. If you concentrate on putting in the order, your production will soon increase.

- Think about your own need to express as well as your baby's need for milk when planning how you will manage separations.

- If you have to be apart from your baby, aim to breastfeed as often as possible when you're with him, to allow him to catch up and to help maintain your milk production.

- Your baby may not need to use a bottle; if he is five months or older when you have to leave him he may prefer a beaker or 'sippy' cup.

- Lots of babies refuse to take milk from anyone other than their mother. They don't starve – they just make up for it with lots of breastfeeds later.

- Planning feeds with your child's carer is an important part of minimising disruption to breastfeeding.

- If you are going back to work, tell your employer in advance you are planning to continue breastfeeding. They are legally obliged to adjust your work commitments to enable you to do this.

10

Six months
and beyond

Breastmilk is all your baby needs for the first six months of her life and you can expect it to remain her main source of nourishment until she is around a year old. However, from the middle of her first year, she'll start to move towards solid foods and family mealtimes. These will gradually take over from breastmilk until, eventually, she stops having milk feeds altogether. This transition usually takes *at least* a year. If you keep following your baby's instincts the move to family meals will go at a pace that is naturally right for her, allowing her to continue having as much milk as she needs, alongside as much (or as little) solid food as she wants. This is called baby-led weaning.

Like baby-led breastfeeding, baby-led weaning relies on your baby's natural instincts and abilities to begin eating solid foods when she is ready. It's very different from the parent-led, stage-by-stage, conventional approach to introducing solids. It's a combination of:

- sharing mealtimes with your baby
- allowing her to set the pace
- trusting her to know what she needs, and
- trusting her to feed herself.

This chapter explains how baby-led weaning works and how you can give your baby the opportunity to include solid foods in her diet when she is ready. It also looks at how you can continue to let her lead the way with breastfeeding as she gets older, so that her last breastfeed happens at a time that is right for her.

Starting solid foods the baby-led way

Learning to eat solid food is a natural and inevitable part of development for any healthy baby – just like crawling, walking and talking. And, like those activities, if it's allowed to it will begin spontaneously, at the right time for each baby.

Most babies' digestive and immune systems are not able to cope with anything other than breastmilk or formula before about six months. If they are given other foods earlier than this they may not be able to digest them fully – and, if they are breastfed, they will tend to take less milk to make room for them. This is why, in the UK and worldwide, solid foods are not recommended before six months. If your four-month-old really *is* hungry she will get more nourishment from extra breastfeeds than she will from other foods.

The skills and co-ordination your baby needs for handling food develop at about the same rate as her need for a more varied diet and the ability of her gut to digest other foods. The traditional signs of readiness for solids that parents have been told to look out for, such as waking at night and watching other people eating, are now known to have nothing to do with needing other foods. They are simply a normal part of a baby's development that start to happen at around four months old. You will know your baby is truly ready when she can sit upright, reach out and grab objects, take them to her mouth and gnaw on them with her gums. In other words, if you give her the opportunity, she will start by herself.

Of course, babies develop at different rates, so some will be reaching for food a week or so before six months, while for others it will be several weeks later. For a rough summary, see *What to expect when*, page 271. The important thing, in a baby-led approach to weaning, is that it should be *your baby's* decision to reach for food, and her decision to take it to her mouth.

Why self feeding makes sense

By the time your baby is ready to start discovering how to eat solid foods she has already developed most of the skills she needs to do it. She has been feeding herself (as opposed to 'being fed') since her very first breastfeed (see Chapter 4) and, because of the way she's used her mouth muscles, she's strengthened them for chewing. She's also been watching you eat, and practising picking things up and taking them to her mouth. And she's been tasting your food through your milk.

Because of this, most babies instinctively want – and are able – to work out how to feed themselves with their fingers. There's no need for spoon feeding. And because by six months they can chew most foods (whether or not they have teeth), there's no need for their food to be pureed. Spoon feeding is appropriate for babies who are not able to feed themselves (those with certain physical disabilities or delayed development, for example) but the vast majority of six-month-olds don't need it.

Breastfed babies are used to controlling how much they eat and how quickly, and whether to have just a drink or a full, fat-rich feed (see page 30), and they can continue to make these decisions when they move on to solid foods. **Allowing babies to feed themselves ensures they eat what they need and don't cut down on breastmilk before they're ready.** It also enables them to learn how to manage different textures confidently and safely. Recent research shows that babies who were introduced to solid foods this way make healthier food choices and may be less prone to obesity in later childhood.

'From the beginning I fed Mia when she wanted. Sometimes she wouldn't feed much and other times she seemed to gorge herself. When it came to solids, of course she had to stay in control – it seemed insane to suddenly start stuffing her full of mush just to make *me* feel better. She eats really well and has however much she needs, just as she always has done. There's no stress at mealtimes; we just sit and eat together. It's great.'

Kirsty, mother of Mia, two years

Will she eat enough food?

Most babies don't actually *eat* any solid food for several weeks after they start handling it. This is normal; they need to learn about tastes and textures, and to practise chewing, before they start to rely on food for nourishment. In a healthy, full-term baby the combination of breastmilk and the nutrients stored in her body while she was in the womb are enough to ensure full nutrition until she's *at least* six months old – and probably until she is eight or nine months.

From six months onwards your baby will begin to need very small amounts of additional nutrients (mainly iron and zinc), which she will get by gradually expanding her diet – but she won't need to eat large quantities; small tastes will be enough. The first sign that your baby has managed to swallow something will probably be when you see 'bits' in her poo, but she will continue to have 'breastfeeding poo' (runny and yellow), with occasional bits, for several months after she has started exploring other foods. Later, as she begins to eat more, her stools will start to become more solid, darker and smellier – especially once she starts to cut down her intake of breastmilk.

At some point – often around eight or nine months – babies seem to make the connection between hunger and solid food. It's then that they begin to eat more purposefully, as though they are actually hungry, and to play with food less. It's likely that this coincides with their growing need for extra nutrition.

Provided your baby has been allowed to handle food as often as she wants, by the time she needs additional nutrients she will be an accomplished eater and able to manage a wide variety of foods, so she will have no problem getting them.

Breastfeeding alongside the introduction of solid foods not only ensures good nutrition, it actually helps with the digestion of those other foods. It's thought the unique ingredients of human milk may also reduce the chances of food allergies and intolerances, such as coeliac disease. Infant formula and 'follow-on' milks cannot provide this sort of protection.

Getting to grips with solid foods

If your baby is given the opportunity to show you when she is ready to begin handling food, she will simply grab some from the table, take it to her mouth and start munching on it. At first she'll have most success with larger pieces of food that she can pick up easily, with some sticking out of her fist. As she becomes more dextrous she'll learn to manage smaller pieces (and eventually progress to using cutlery).

Your baby's motivation to try solid foods is not hunger. After all, she doesn't yet know that food can fill her tummy. She is driven by curiosity and her instinct to develop new skills. She will experiment with food just as she does with a new toy, exploring it with her hands and her mouth, squishing, smearing and licking it and discovering what it can do. Gradually she'll learn to bite pieces off with her gums and work out how to chew them. As long as she is sitting upright, the first few times she does this the food will fall out of her mouth. Then, when she has developed the ability to move chewed food to the back of her mouth, some will be swallowed.

It's better, in the early days, if your baby *isn't* hungry when you offer her the chance to handle food. If she is, she'll get frustrated – just as she would if you tried to interest her in a new toy when all she wanted was a breastfeed. Mealtimes are playtimes in the beginning; if your baby is hungry or thirsty, it's your breast she needs.

What happens with breastfeeding?

For the first few months after she starts solid food anything your baby eats will be *in addition to* her milk and breastfeeding will carry on much as before. Then, some time around nine months, she'll begin gradually to need less breastmilk. However, unless she is having other drinks (which would decrease her need for breastmilk as a drink), the number of breastfeeds she asks for probably won't change noticeably at first; she will simply carry on asking for them in her usual way but take slightly less milk at each feed. In time, you'll notice that she asks for some milk feeds a little later than usual, especially after a meal where she's eaten quite a lot of solid food. Then, when she is regularly eating and drinking at mealtimes, she may decide to skip some breastfeeds altogether, turning away when she's offered the breast. All you need to do is to respond to her cues, just as you have until now.

Even if you notice a fairly consistent drop in breastfeeding, it may not be a permanent change. It's common for babies to go back to breastfeeding more often and lose interest in solid foods for short periods, especially when they are teething or fighting off an infection. They may want nothing but breastmilk for a week or two, then switch back to eating solid foods and taking less milk. Babies also tend to want to breastfeed more often when they are feeling emotionally unsettled. If you go back to work (see page 156), move house or go on holiday, for instance, you can expect your baby to ask for more breastfeeds to help her cope with the change, whether or not she is eating much solid food.

If your baby's appetite for milk gets less but then suddenly increases again, your breasts will adapt within a day or two – even if your milk production has already gone down

Baby-led weaning at a glance

How to start:

- As soon as your baby can sit up with little or no support, start including her in your mealtimes and snacks whenever possible. Choose times when your baby is not hungry or sleepy.
- Make sure the food you are eating is healthy, so your baby can share it and copy you as you eat.
- Prepare for some mess. Lots of food will go on the floor to start with. A clean splash mat under the chair means you can re-offer food that has been dropped. A plate is not necessary at first and may be a distraction.
- Sit your baby on your lap or in a highchair. Make sure she is sitting upright and that she can reach the table or tray easily.
- Let her share the food on your plate, or put a few pieces of food in front of her for her to pick up (babies can be overwhelmed by too much choice).
- Offer your baby water to drink with her meals – but don't be surprised if she isn't interested. She may prefer to continue to have all her drinks at the breast.
- Continue to offer breastfeeds on demand.

Foods to offer:

- Prepare nutritious food so that your baby can pick it up easily – thick sticks of vegetables, about 5 to 8cm (2 to 3½ in) long, pieces of fruit, strips of meat and fingers of toast are all suitable to start with.
- Include new shapes and textures gradually, so that your baby has the chance to practise and develop her skills. Rice, minced meat, and runny, crunchy or slippery foods all provide an interesting challenge.
- Aim for a variety of flavours. Babies don't need bland food (many strong flavours will be familiar to her from your breastmilk).

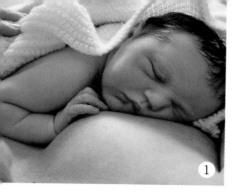
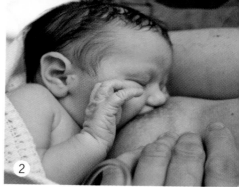

▲ As soon as she's born, Scarlett is laid skin to skin on her mother's chest. She rests a while, then finds the breast and has her first feed.

Mike helps Billie to hold their newborn twins, Ottilie and Anna, in skin contact, so they can feed as soon as they're ready (see page 22). ▼

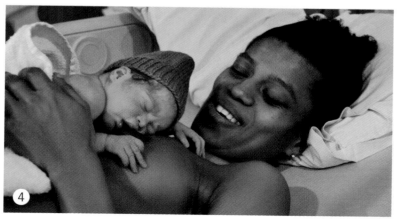

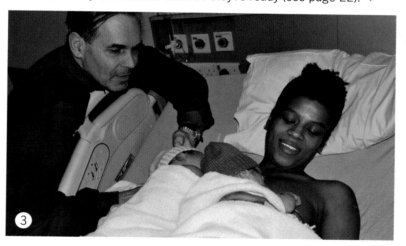

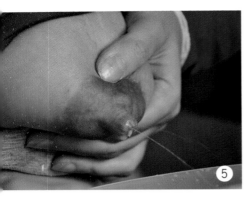

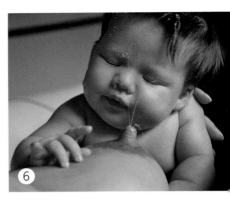

▲ Hand expressing breastmilk is a useful skill and is easy once you get the knack (see page 86).

▲ Artemis is able to pull herself away from a strong let-down reflex (see page 24). She'll wait a few seconds for the flow to subside before she goes back on to the breast.

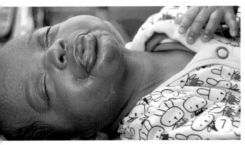

◄ Munira has finished feeding and now looks 'milk drunk'.

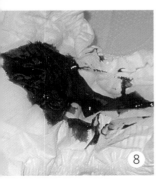

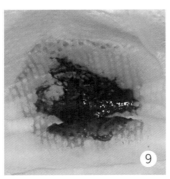

▲ These photos show a newborn baby's poo on the first, third and fifth days after birth. The gradual change from the greenish black, sticky meconium to yellow, runny poo shows that she is getting plenty of milk (see page 98).

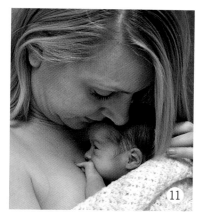

Michaela holds Jacob, one of her premature twins, in kangaroo care (see page 193). Being held this way has many benefits and allows him to breastfeed as soon as he's ready.

Trudy holds newborn Noah in skin-to-skin contact on the operating table after his Caesarean birth, with Derek looking on. Skin contact is the best way for breastfeeding to begin and is especially important after this type of birth (see page 63). ▼

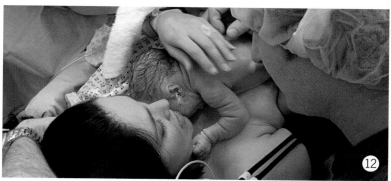

If you have a blocked duct or mastitis your baby can help to clear it by feeding in a position that targets the sore area (see page 239). Leaning over your baby to feed is especially helpful.

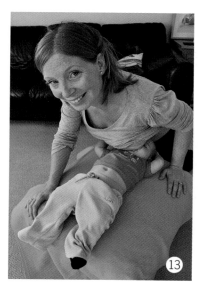

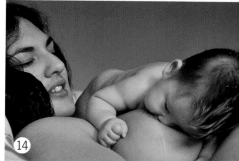

Beatrice, six weeks, approaches the breast, nose to nipple, and scoops up a big mouthful, with the nipple pointing towards the roof of her mouth. Once attached, her chin is pressing into the breast, her nose is free, her cheeks are full, and more of her mother's areola is visible above her top lip than below her bottom lip (see page 50). When she's finished feeding she lets go of the breast and sleeps.

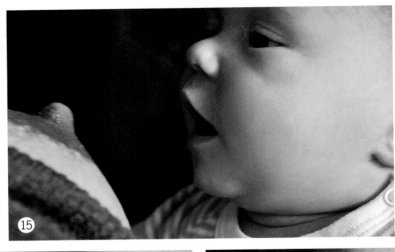

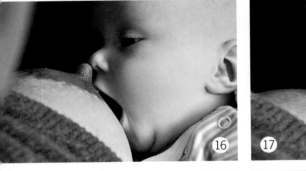

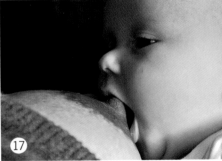

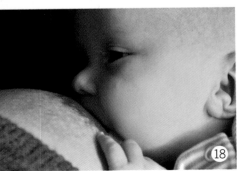

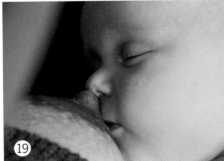

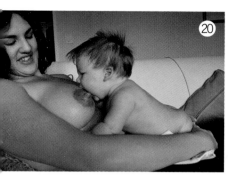

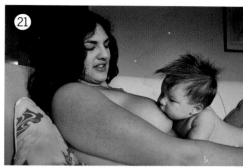

Artemis, eight weeks, shows how easily she can use her instincts when she's lying on her mother (see page 37). Her head and arms are strong enough for her to get into a position where she can easily attach, and she uses her hands to steady herself and the breast. She doesn't need any help!

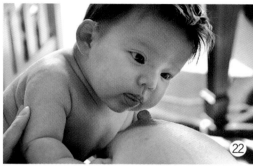

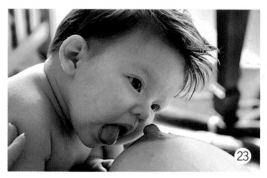

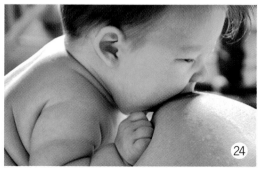

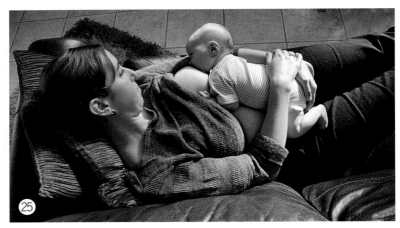

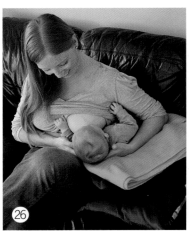

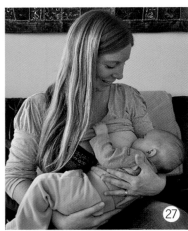

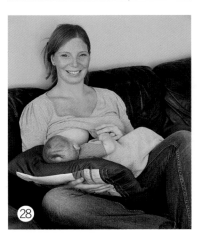

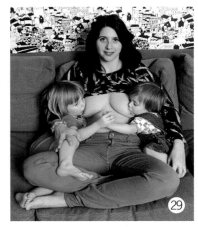

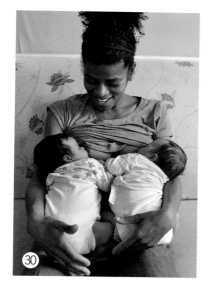

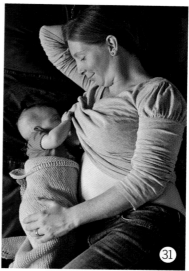

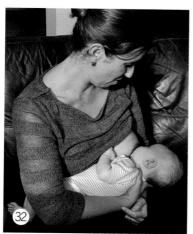

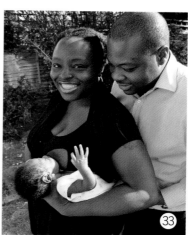

Whether you're feeding one baby or two, as long as they are in a position that makes it easy for them to feed, you can sit, stand, lie back or lie down to breastfeed – whatever suits you and your baby (or babies).

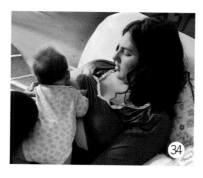

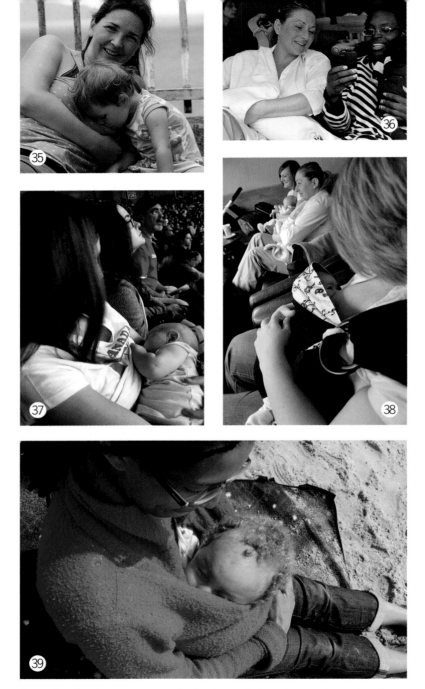

Breastfeeding is an easy way to feed your baby when you're out and about. If you want, you can use your clothes, a sling or a muslin to cover up with.

Unless there are allergies in your family there is no need to start with one taste at a time.

- Avoid salt, ready-meals, junk food and additives as much as possible (you may need to check labels carefully – some common foods, such as baked beans and gravy, can be very high in salt). Honey and undercooked eggs carry a small risk of food poisoning, so they should be avoided until your baby is over a year old.

What to expect:

- Mealtimes are for learning and experimenting, at first, so your baby probably won't eat much for the first few months. Provided she can breastfeed whenever she wants, breastmilk will continue to provide all her nourishment.
- Many babies gag on food in the early weeks. This is a normal protective reflex to push food forward, away from the airway, while they are learning how to manage it. The gag reflex is more sensitive in babies than adults and is triggered further forward on the tongue. It's *not* the same as choking and it doesn't seem to bother babies. Once the food has been pushed forward, either it falls out of their mouth or they carry on chewing it.

Remember to:

- Keep mealtimes enjoyable – let your baby play and don't hurry her or try to persuade her to eat more than she wants.
- Trust your baby to cut down her milk feeds whenever she is ready.
- Explain how baby-led weaning works to anyone involved in feeding your baby.

Safety:

- Make sure your baby is sitting upright to eat, not leaning back in a bouncy chair, or slumping forwards or sideways. This will allow her to control the food in her mouth safely.

- Don't put anything in your baby's mouth for her – and don't let anyone else do so either (watch out for 'helpful' toddlers).
- Don't offer your baby hard nuts (in pieces or whole); remove stones from food such as olives and cherries; cut small round fruits, such as grapes, in half.
- Never leave your baby alone with food.

See *Sources of information and support*, page 278, for where to get more information on baby-led weaning.

considerably. If you let her feed as much as she wants your supply will soon catch up.

Babies rarely stop breastfeeding of their own accord before their first birthday. If your baby is under a year old and turns down the offer of a feed lots of times in a row, don't assume she's ready to give up the breast. It's more likely she's going through a nursing strike (see page 124). She'll probably go back to breastfeeding within a few days if you continue to offer her the opportunity.

Breastfeeding as your child grows older

Breastfeeding doesn't have to end just because your baby is no longer relying on it for her nourishment – it can carry on for several more years, if you both want. The World Health Organization recommends that all babies should be breastfed for at least two years but there isn't an upper age limit. Many young children continue feeding two or three times a day – perhaps first thing in the morning and last thing at night, plus odd times when they fall over or are tired or upset – well into early childhood. And continuing to breastfeed will benefit *your* health, too (see page 8).

Many women expect to stop breastfeeding by the time their child reaches a certain age. Sometimes this is because they are unaware that it's normal for children to continue to breastfeed into their second, third or fourth year – perhaps because breastfeeding at this age usually happens at home and is rarely talked about. However, many of those who had planned to stop breastfeeding after, for instance, a year or 18 months, find, when the time comes, that they no longer want to stop. If both you and your child are enjoying this special time together there's no need for it to end. Stopping before one of you is ready can be challenging (see *Ending breastfeeding – who decides?*, page 176); it's easier to carry on until the time feels right for you both.

'I haven't made a decision to carry on breastfeeding Celia – but the decision to stop will be hers. Sometimes I've thought I'll stop soon but it's never felt right just to take it away from her. At night she has a couple of sucks to get to sleep. In the morning we'll spend a good hour feeding if we have the time. It's becoming gradually less and less. A year ago there's no way she would have said no if I offered a feed, but now she says no sometimes. She'll stop when she's ready – I'm in no hurry.'

Miranda, mother of Celia, two years

Many people assume that, once a baby is having a good, varied diet of solid foods, there's no value in breastmilk. This isn't true. **The protective factors in your milk will continue to help your child to resist infections for as long as you continue to feed her.** As she starts to drink less and your production winds down, your milk will become gradually more concentrated – almost like colostrum again – giving her an extra boost of immunity as she faces the rough and tumble of childhood. In fact, a child's immune system is not fully mature until she is about six years old, so it's reasonable to suppose that children can continue to benefit from the antibodies in breastmilk until they are well past toddlerhood.

Breastmilk doesn't lose its nutritional properties just because the child is eating other foods. It continues to provide balanced nutrition and is the single most complete food available to humans. Research has shown that children who stop breastfeeding before two years of age have a greater risk of illness and take longer to recover than those who feed for longer. Continuing to breastfeed means you will always have a nourishing, easy-to-digest food to give your child if she becomes ill, and many mothers keep breastfeeding through the toddler years for this reason alone.

However, feeding a toddler is very different from feeding a newborn, so you may need to make some adjustments to the way breastfeeding happens to enable you and your child to carry on enjoying this part of your relationship.

Toddlers aren't always discreet!

By the time your baby reaches her first birthday she'll be very quick and efficient at breastfeeding, and able to latch on from virtually any angle. However, as she grows in confidence and dexterity you may find that she asks for feeds in ways that you don't really like.

Toddlers want to exert their independence and show everyone what they can do. They don't understand that their mother may not want them to start helping themselves to her breast – by pulling up her top and grabbing at her bra – when they are in a café or at the bus stop. So you may want to give your child some guidance on how you'd like her to behave when she wants a feed.

Many mothers have a word for breastfeeding that they use from very early on when they offer their baby a feed – 'booby' or 'mummy milk', for example. If you are likely to be embarrassed when your baby learns to talk and starts asking for 'booby', you may want to opt for a more neutral word from the outset. You can then encourage her to ask for a feed quietly, using her special word, rather than announcing her intentions loudly (or just helping herself). Some women choose a word that won't mean anything to anyone else (except perhaps another breastfeeding mother) – 'noo-noo', for example. Others use a phrase such as 'mummy hug', 'sleepy hug' or 'special cuddle', which won't raise any eyebrows.

As she gets older your child will begin to be able to wait a little while to feed. This will be useful if you are in a place where you don't feel comfortable feeding her. You'll find you can distract her so that she forgets for a while or, if she's old enough, simply tell her, when she asks, that she can have milk later.

Dealing with negative opinions

Many people don't know about the benefits of breastfeeding past babyhood and they may feel uncomfortable about toddlers and young children being breastfed. For the generation of parents (now grandparents and great-grandparents) who were encouraged to get their child to do everything early (solids by three months, no milk feeds past a year, and so on) it can be especially puzzling.

You will probably find it useful to have a few strategies to help you deal with awkward questions and unsupportive comments. For example, you could explain the reasons why breastfeeding is beneficial for small children (the UNICEF UK Baby Friendly Initiative website is useful; see *Sources of information and support*, page 278). Or you may prefer to say that health professionals advise breastfeeding for as long as possible. Alternatively, you could simply take the line that you don't need to justify your breastfeeding relationship with your child to anyone, and change the subject.

You may find it helpful to make contact with other mothers who are breastfeeding older babies and children, perhaps through a group such as La Leche League. See page 121 and

Sources of information and support, page 278, for details of breastfeeding groups and helplines.

Breastfeeding during pregnancy and beyond

Many women become pregnant again while they are still breastfeeding their older child (although, when breastfeeding is baby-led, it's unusual for a mother to become pregnant again within six months – see page 136) and there is rarely a reason why it is not safe for them to continue. Women who are prone to miscarriage or premature birth are occasionally advised to stop breastfeeding for part of their pregnancy but, in general, a mother's body is perfectly able to nourish two babies at the same time.

Breastfeeding when you're pregnant

Some mothers find that breastfeeding continues smoothly throughout their next pregnancy but most notice changes as their body prepares for a new arrival. Mother and baby can usually find ways of adapting their technique to accommodate what is happening (see below), but occasionally the changes mean that breastfeeding has to end early.

The most obvious cause of disruption to breastfeeding is the growing 'bump'. This may make some of your usual breastfeeding positions uncomfortable or impossible. If you can, explain to your child that your tummy is tender and enlist her help to find a position that works for both of you.

Another common problem is increased tenderness of the nipples, which can make breastfeeding painful – either for a few weeks or, in some cases, for most of the pregnancy. Negotiating shorter breastfeeds with your child, and making sure she doesn't 'play' with your other nipple or keep coming on and off the breast may make feeding more tolerable.

The other key change is to the breastmilk itself. Although some women carry on making large quantities of milk throughout their pregnancy, most find that their breasts revert to producing colostrum, ready for the new baby. This changes the taste and consistency of the milk, and the amount available – any of which is likely to be noticed by the breastfeeding child. A simple explanation may be enough to help your child cope with this development but she may decide that she prefers not to breastfeed, at least temporarily.

Some toddlers decide to wean themselves off the breast while their mother is pregnant and then want to start feeding again when the new baby arrives. If you are prepared for this to happen, and welcome it, your child is less likely to feel rejected in favour of the new arrival.

'When I was pregnant with Charlie my breasts were so tender I had to clamp my jaws together whenever Grace fed. But I wanted her to decide when she was ready to stop and I wanted her and the new baby to feed together. Then one night she latched on and said: "Mummy, no milk." I don't know if there wasn't any or she didn't want any. I was relieved, but sad that I wouldn't be tandem feeding. But a few months after Charlie was born she asked to try it again, so I did it after all.'

Jade, mother of Grace, two years, and Charlie, nine months

Whether or not your toddler is still breastfeeding near the end of your pregnancy, she won't have forgotten about it. However, she won't automatically know that new babies need to do it, so if she's old enough to understand it's important to explain this to her. It may help to show her pictures of herself as a baby, and to point out that newborns can't eat all the other sorts of food that she enjoys, which means they need to drink lots of breastmilk. Taking her to visit a friend who is breastfeeding a young baby (or to a breastfeeding support group) may help her to understand that new babies need to breastfeed often, rather than just occasionally.

You can breastfeed your baby and your older child

Breastfeeding siblings who are different in age (or 'tandem' feeding) can be one of the best ways of preventing an older brother or sister feeling rejected or jealous of a new baby. For many women it happens naturally, especially if there's not much gap between their pregnancies, while others plan to tandem feed specifically to ease the transition for their older child. However, some negotiation may be needed to ensure that the new baby gets what she needs.

In the first few days, if your older child wants to feed at around the same time as her new sibling, it's best to ask her to wait, just to be sure the new baby gets her share of colostrum. The exception to this is if you are still producing large volumes of milk; in this case allowing your toddler to feed first will help to lessen the flow and make it easier for your new baby to manage. **Including both baby and child in breastfeeding will encourage your milk production to increase rapidly, so there will soon be plenty for two.** (Expect your toddler to have a brief bout of loose stools, brought on by drinking colostrum.)

Holding a toddler and a new baby so they can feed at the same time can present a challenge. In the first few weeks, the easiest way for you to feed your children together may be lying back on your bed, with your new baby on top of you and your toddler next to you. If you prefer to sit up, try asking your toddler to sit or kneel (or stand) beside you to feed, to give you more room to position your little one.

If you are used to a toddler pretty much helping herself at the breast, you may be surprised to rediscover how much support a newborn needs and how long it takes her to feed. Giving your new baby the time she needs to work out how to latch on while you have an older child wanting to share you may not be easy. Some mothers enlist their older child's help to show her sibling what to do, while others insist that she allow the new baby to feed separately or to get started first, before she joins in.

It's common for older children to want to negotiate which breast is 'theirs'. While it will usually be possible to feed your new baby exclusively from the breast that her sibling has allocated to her, if she is taking a while to get the hang of breastfeeding you may have to ask your older child to feed from that breast, too, to ensure both breasts are 'asked' to make plenty of milk.

Toddlers can be very erratic about how often they want to breastfeed. For the first few weeks after the baby's birth, while your milk production is unsettled, your breasts may become overfull at times, making it difficult for your newborn to attach and putting you at risk of engorgement or mastitis. Encouraging some consistency in your toddler's feeding pattern will help to keep things on an even keel. Of course, if your breasts do become uncomfortable, your older child is the ideal person to help relieve them.

Tandem feeding, even when planned, can sometimes be difficult emotionally for the mother, especially in the first week or so. You may be surprised to find your protective instincts for your newborn kicking in suddenly, so much so that you even feel resentful towards your older child when she wants to feed. This is entirely normal, and is nature's way of ensuring that the most vulnerable member of the family is cared for. But it may mean that the transition to tandem feeding isn't quite as seamless as you'd envisaged. And if these emotions coincide with your older child feeling left out and demanding more of your attention, life could become fraught. Sharing your feelings with your partner or with another mother who has tandem fed may help (if you don't know anyone to talk to you may find an online forum or the La Leche League helpline useful – see *Sources of information and support*, page 278). Having special time alone with each child, and remembering how much your older child may need the emotional reassurance of breastfeeding at this time, can also help.

'Tandem feeding was hard at first. The new baby latching on was like learning how to breastfeed all over again and Micky wanted milk at the same time. Sometimes it would be easier to feed Micky first. Toddlers often need just a little to be satisfied – it's more about comfort and knowing they can still have the breast, and he was so needy because of the new baby.'

Sharon, mother of Micky, four years, and Carly, two years

If one of your children is poorly, both you and the other child will already have been exposed to any germs so you needn't change the way you feed them. If the older one has an infection, the antibodies in your milk will help to prevent your newborn becoming ill – or help her to recover quickly – and will also help your toddler to get well faster. The only exception to this is if either child gets an infection of the mouth (such as thrush, see page 232). In that case, if you spot the problem early, allocating them one breast each may help to prevent the other child (and breast) developing the condition – although you should still treat both breasts and both children.

Ending breastfeeding – who decides?

In many cases breastfeeding ends naturally, as the child outgrows her need for it. In others, the mother makes the decision to stop. However, it's rare for babies who've been allowed to set the pace with weaning to be ready to manage without milk feeds before they are at least a year old. **If you have to (or choose to) stop breastfeeding when your baby is under 12 months, you'll need to give her formula.** See page 224 for how to replace breastfeeds with formula, and for what to do if you need or want to stop breastfeeding quickly.

When the end of breastfeeding is chosen by the child it can be either quite sudden or a gradual process. Some children

FEELING UNDER PRESSURE TO STOP

Sometimes mothers feel under pressure from their partners, family or friends to stop breastfeeding. But giving up something you're enjoying may be very hard emotionally – for you and your child. Stopping when neither of you is truly ready may make family life miserable and could lead to resentment.

announce that they don't want to feed any more; others continue to have one feed a day until something, such as a holiday, changes the usual routine and the breastfeed gets forgotten. Even when it seems as though your toddler has had her last breastfeed, she may surprise you by asking to feed again two weeks later.

Breastfeeding doesn't always end at a time that both mother and child are happy with. Sometimes the mother is ready to stop before her child has got to that point; in other cases it's the mother who finds it difficult to accept her child's decision to stop breastfeeding. If you and your child (over a year old) aren't ready for breastfeeding to end at the same time you may find the suggestions below helpful for working things out.

What if I want to stop but my child doesn't?

Some mothers want to stop breastfeeding because they 'want their body back' or because a new chapter is opening in their life – a new pregnancy, for example, or a new job. Although breastfeeding does not have to end in these circumstances, you may choose to leave it behind as part of this transition.

If you are simply fed up with your child asking for milk at awkward times, perhaps all you need to do is to cut her feeding back gradually (see below) until she is having only a couple of feeds a day – maybe bedtime and morning – then reassess how you feel. It may be that you simply need to be feeding less, rather than not at all.

If you *do* want to stop but your child wants to continue, be prepared for the process to take several weeks. She needs time to come to terms with what is happening and your breasts need time to decrease production gradually. Try to avoid periods that are likely to be emotionally unsettling for her, such as around her starting nursery or the arrival of a new baby, and be ready to put things on hold if she is upset or poorly. Remember that even if breastfeeding is driving *you* mad, your child may still love it and feel rejected and confused when you want to take it away.

Helping your child to give up the breast

There are several strategies you can choose from to bring about the end of breastfeeding for a baby over a year old.

- *Don't offer, don't refuse.* Rather than offer feeds when your child would normally want them, simply wait for her to ask. If it turns out that she was ready to stop feeding anyway, this method may be very quick, in which case you may find yourself offering the occasional feed after all so that you don't have to express to stay comfortable.

- *Distraction.* When you sense that your child is about to ask for a feed, suggest a distraction, such as a game or a trip to the shops. This can work very well for daytime feeds, especially at a time when there are lots of exciting activities, such as when you are on holiday. Distracting your child *before* she asks to feed, rather than trying to divert her when she has already decided that's what she needs, will prevent her becoming distressed.

- *Make yourself unavailable.* Get your partner or someone else to take over your child's care at key times (such as bedtime) for a while. If necessary, arrange to be out of the house (perhaps by inventing an urgent errand). Make sure she is still having plenty of cuddles from you at other times. If she usually needs to feed to help her doze off for a nap, a drive in the car or (if she is still small enough) a walk in the buggy or sling may work instead.

- *Negotiate a date with your child* (for instance, her next birthday, Christmas, Easter or the first/last day of an exciting holiday), then cut out breastfeeds gradually, working towards that date. This can work well with an older child, who is able to understand the concept of time. Don't insist on the earliest possible date – it's important that your child feels she's agreed to the plan. Be prepared to renegotiate if she changes her mind when the time comes.

- *Planned schedule.* This approach only really works if your child's breastfeeding pattern is fairly consistent from day to day. Just cut out one feed at a time, allowing a few days in between for your breasts to adjust. To minimise discomfort, try to keep the gaps between remaining feeds as even as possible. Expect her to resist losing the last feed more strongly than the others.

Whichever approach you choose, make sure you have plenty of healthy snacks and drinks on hand for times when your child is likely to be hungry or thirsty. You may also find it helpful to minimise reminders that could trigger a request to feed; for example, by opting for a trip to the park when you'd normally be cuddled up feeding on the sofa, wearing perfume to mask the smell of your milk and choosing tops with no easy access to your breasts.

Night-time feeds are likely to be the last to go and they can be the hardest to stop. One idea (if your child is old enough to understand) is to say goodnight at bedtime to all the different things that have to go to sleep at night: the birds, the sun, your child's friends – and your breasts, so that she doesn't expect them to be available if she wakes. However, it's rare that stopping night-time breastfeeds means that a child stops waking during the night; you may find it takes you slightly longer to comfort your child when that happens, without breastfeeding to soothe her back to sleep. Some mothers are happy to keep night-time feeds going long after daytime feeds have stopped, for this reason.

> 'I had to stop feeding Ryan when he was two for medical reasons. It was hard. Feeds during the day went first, because he was easily distracted. But every morning he'd wake up and say "Milk, Mummy", and he'd feed. Then, eventually one morning he said "Porridge". The night feed went after that – I told him to say goodbye to feeding and his dad put him to bed. The whole thing took several months. With Jamie, my youngest, I wanted him to feed for as long as possible but he decided himself just before his third birthday. We were sitting on the sofa and he was having a feed, he came off and just looked at it and walked away. I knew then that it was his last feed. There was no real warning – I was gutted.'
>
> Natalie, *mother of Ryan, six years, and Jamie, three years*

What if my child wants to stop but I don't?

Sometimes women find their child has had enough of the breast long before they expected them to. If you have read all about the nutritional, immunological and emotional benefits of feeding a child for several years but your toddler decides she can do without it, this can be bitterly disappointing. Many mothers mourn the passing of the special closeness of their breastfeeding relationship, especially if it has ended suddenly.

It's impossible to persuade a child to breastfeed when they don't want to because *they* have to do the feeding – all you do is provide the breast. So if your child decides to stop feeding there will probably be little you can do to change her mind. However, the following may be worth a try:

- If your child uses a dummy or has a bottle, these may be satisfying her need to suck; discouraging their use may tempt her back to the breast.
- Continuing to offer her the chance to feed at times when she used to particularly enjoy it, such as at bedtime, or when she is tired or upset, may rekindle her interest.
- Some of the suggestions for overcoming a nursing strike (see page 126), such as sharing a bath with your child, may remind her what she is missing.

Generally, be available for her, but don't nag her to feed – it's unlikely to win her over.

If you feel your child has stopped breastfeeding before you would have liked, it may help to remind yourself that baby-led breastfeeding is about trusting your child's decisions throughout – including her ability to know when her need for breastfeeding is over. She is still young and will continue to need plenty of mummy time.

Key points

- At around six months your baby is likely to be ready to begin experimenting with solid foods. Her natural instincts and abilities will make it easy for her to feed herself.

- If you offer your baby the chance to join in with healthy family meals she will show you when she is ready to share your food.

- If your baby is allowed to decide how much solid food to eat, she will cut down her milk feeds gradually, at a pace that is right for her.

- Breastfeeding beyond one year is normal and natural – babies under a year old are very unlikely to stop breastfeeding of their own accord.

- Many children carry on breastfeeding once or twice a day for several years. Breastmilk never loses its protective properties and breastfeeding is one of the best ways to comfort a young child.

- You may want to work out with your toddler some discreet ways for her to ask to feed.

- If you want to you can continue to breastfeed when you are pregnant – and carry on feeding your older child when the new baby arrives.

- Ideally, breastfeeding will come to a natural conclusion when you and your child are both ready. If it has to happen earlier than this there are strategies you can employ to help you both make the adjustment.

part III

Less common situations

11

Premature babies and multiples

Babies often come early and they sometimes come in pairs, threes or more. Having a baby born prematurely, or having more than one baby (whether or not they are born early), brings all sorts of challenges for parents but it doesn't mean breastfeeding isn't possible, or that it can't be at least partly baby-led. This chapter looks at how to recognise your baby's (or babies') abilities and make the most of them, so that together you can benefit from the unique start that breastfeeding brings.

Breastfeeding when your baby is born early

When a baby is born early, all previous plans go out of the window. Nothing quite prepares you for the shock of becoming a parent earlier than you originally anticipated and the support of people who understand what you're going through can be invaluable. (See *Sources of information and support*, page 278, for details of organisations that offer support to parents of premature babies.)

Depending on how premature he is, your little one may need to be cared for in either a neonatal unit (NNU, also sometimes called a special care baby unit) or a neonatal intensive care unit (NICU). He may have wires attached to him to monitor his heart rate and oxygen levels, he may have an intravenous drip and a tube through his nose or mouth into his stomach, and he may need help to breathe. And, of course, since premature births are often accompanied by illness in the mother, and/or by some sort of instrumental delivery, you may not be fully well or mobile yourself.

Why breastmilk is important for premature babies

Breastmilk is even more important for your baby if he is born prematurely than it would be if he had arrived on time. This is because his gut is more immature (and less able to tolerate formula milk) and his vulnerability to infection even greater than if he had stayed a bit longer in the womb. In fact, breastmilk is so important for a premature baby's health, both immediately and long term, that many staff who work in neonatal units think of breastmilk as primarily a medicine rather than a food.

Many larger hospitals (and some community health services) have a breastmilk 'bank' that collects and stores donated breastmilk so that it is available for babies who might otherwise have to have formula. But, whenever possible, the ideal milk for a premature baby is his own mother's milk, and especially her colostrum. The best thing you can do for your newborn premature baby is to provide him with your milk from the very beginning.

However, a premature birth presents several challenges in terms of getting breastfeeding up and running and you'll find you are faced with two main obstacles:

- You and your baby are likely to be separated. This may be only briefly or it may be for long periods of time, perhaps extending over several months. Skin-to-skin contact may not be possible for hours, days or even weeks after the birth. And, if your baby has to stay in hospital, privacy will be hard to come by.

- Your baby may be too weak or immature to breastfeed, at first.

Expressing milk for your premature baby

If your baby is premature he may not be able to breastfeed straight away and may not even be ready for milk feeds. But although he'll be getting all his nourishment via an intravenous drip, he will still benefit from your colostrum. A few drops spread around the inside of his mouth will help to protect him from infections, start to strengthen his digestive tract and help him to recognise your taste and smell. You can provide your milk for him – by expressing – as soon as he's born. (You'll find information on expressing breastmilk on pages 86 and Chapter 9.)

Expressing your milk as soon as possible after the birth is also enormously important to set your breasts up for long-term milk production. When a baby is born on time it's the messages the breasts receive during the first two weeks (and especially the first few days) that determine how much milk the mother is able to make in the future (see Chapter 2). But when a baby arrives early, much of what would normally happen to trigger milk production isn't possible. So to ensure plenty of milk, both now and later, you'll need to mimic the frequent feeding your baby would have done if he he'd been born closer to his due date.

The key to getting milk production going by expressing is to start early and do it often. If you can express intensively over the first two weeks (see below), you'll give your breasts a huge 'wake-up' call and your chances of being able to breastfeed your baby for as long as you want will be vastly increased. Your breasts will need this extra stimulation even if your baby is managing to have some of his feeds at the breast, because he won't have the strength or the appetite to put in a big enough order on his own. Make sure your partner and family understand how important this time is so they can give you the support you need to focus on expressing.

Because of the intensive nature of expressing for a premature baby, the hospital staff will make sure you have access to an electric breast pump while you're there. You may also be able to borrow one of their pumps to use at home, or you can hire one from a breastfeeding support organisation (see page 278). Many mothers find these pumps very useful after the first few days. However, colostrum comes in very small amounts and is quite sticky, so hand expression (see page 86) is a much better way to collect this first milk. If someone can sit with you and draw it up in a little syringe as you express it, your baby will be sure to get every drop.

'Frankie was seven weeks premature and was in an incubator for two weeks. It was really hard to express at first – it felt like there was nothing there. They showed me how to hand express, so I had milk ready for him once he was off the drip. I used to set my alarm so I could do it every three hours, day and night. After 10 days I started feeding him myself but it took him about two weeks to open his mouth properly – he used to suck as if my breast was a straw. I was in agony – every night I'd swear I'd give up – then in the morning I'd change my mind. I fed him until he was 10 months but now I wish I'd fed him for longer.'

Kerry, mother of Ella, eight, Joshua, six, and Frankie, 14 months

The NNU staff will be able to guide you on what containers to use for your milk and how to store it. All the equipment needs to be sterile because premature babies are especially vulnerable to infection. Ideally, your baby should have your milk as soon as possible after you've expressed it; if it needs to be refrigerated or frozen, it should be given to him in the order it was expressed – at least in the first couple of weeks

– so you'll need to label each batch clearly with the time you expressed it, as well as the date. (Where possible, fresh milk is always preferable to refrigerated or frozen milk, because some of the protective ingredients are de-activated by cold.)

How to give your breasts a two-week 'wake-up call'

The more you stimulate your breasts to make milk in the first two weeks, the easier breastfeeding will be from then on. Here's what to do:

- If you and your baby are well enough, spend as long as you can immediately after the birth with him lying against your tummy and chest, skin to skin. Hold him like this as often as possible over the next few weeks.
- Start expressing as soon as you can after your baby is born – within an hour is good. If you don't feel well enough to do it yourself, ask your partner or a midwife to do it for you. Hand expressing is best at this stage.
- **Express as often as you can, day and night. Aim for 12 times in 24 hours** – certainly no fewer than eight. The intervals between sessions don't need to be regular – just fit them in whenever you can.
- Try to avoid long gaps – four hours during the day (or six hours at night) should be the absolute maximum. Plan ahead: if you know you're going to need a gap of more than two or three hours, see if you can fit in some extra expressing before and afterwards. If you are in a place where you can't save the milk, express anyway and throw it away. You'll have more milk in the long run if you keep putting in the order.
- Use some of the tips on page 147 to get your oxytocin flowing before and during each expressing session. If you can't be near your baby, close your eyes and visualise yourself holding him, stroking him, smelling

him and kissing him. Try to include a few minutes of breast massage at every session. If you can be with your baby but can't hold him, ask the NNU staff to help you to get some privacy near him for expressing – for instance by putting a screen around you both – to make it easier to get your milk flowing.

- Use hand expression or a pump, whichever you prefer. Ideally, use hand expression while the amounts are small and move on to a combination of hand and pump as the volume increases, starting and finishing each session with hand expression.

- If you're using a pump, make sure the funnel is the right size for you, so that it compresses your milk ducts effectively. Ask the staff for help with this, and don't be afraid to experiment with larger or smaller funnels to find the one that suits you.

- Start each pumping session with the pump on a low setting and increase the rate and strength gradually, as the milk starts to flow. There is no need to aim for maximum power; just find the level that works best for you.

- When the milk stops flowing with a pump, do a bit of breast massage and then some hand expression. This will usually trigger another let-down reflex. Then go back to the pump. When the flow subsides again, wait a couple of minutes and have another go. You'll be surprised how much extra milk you can get this way.

- Keep expressing for as long as you are getting milk out. Switch to the second breast when the flow subsides on the first, then go back to the first one again, then the second. Better still, express from both breasts at the same time (this is possible using a pump as well as by hand – ask the hospital staff for help).

- You may want to use breast compression (see page 196) while expressing, to help you get more milk.

TIP

If you're expressing long term you may occasionally experience a dip in how much milk you get when you express. This could be because your let-down reflex isn't working as well as it was (maybe you're worried about your baby's condition, or maybe you've started to take the reflex for granted and have cut down on the preliminaries you use at the beginning of an expressing session), or it may simply be because you haven't been expressing very often recently. Taking your time to get ready to express, and fitting in a couple of extra expressing sessions a day, is probably all that's needed to boost your milk supply again.

- **Focus on putting in the order, not on what you're getting out.** Don't be disheartened if you just get small amounts to start with. It can take a little while, but the more you 'ask for', the more you'll start to get.

After the 'wake-up'

If you follow this approach, by the end of the two weeks you'll be producing lots of milk – probably over 500ml per day, and possibly as much as 750ml or more. Of course, your baby won't need this much for a while yet but you will have given your breasts a very clear message about what they need to do. If your baby is still not ready to have all his feeds at your breast you'll need to keep expressing, though not quite as intensively. With a bit of experimentation you'll find a pattern that keeps you producing milk fairly steadily. Once your baby is having most of his feeds directly from your breast, you'll be able to phase out the expressing altogether.

Hindmilk feeding – helping your baby to get more of the fattier milk

If you are producing more milk than your baby needs the NNU staff may suggest that you do something called 'hindmilk feeding', so that he gets the maximum calories in the minimum of volume. At each expressing session (or feed) your milk gets gradually creamier and more full of calories as the fat content increases. This fattier milk is sometimes known as 'hindmilk'. Hindmilk feeding ensures that the baby gets the calorie-rich milk first. Here's how it works:

- You express some milk from each breast (about half the amount you usually get) into one container and set it aside.
- You then express the remaining milk from both breasts into a second container. (It will probably look visibly creamier than the first batch.)
- Your baby is given the *second* lot of milk first, followed by as much of the first as he needs to complete his feed.

You may also be advised that your milk needs to be 'fortified'. This involves the addition of some extra minerals (for example, calcium), usually as a powder. It doesn't mean your milk is not good quality – it's just a nutritional safety net that is thought to be important for very premature babies.

Feeding your baby before he is ready to breastfeed

Most babies are not mature enough to feed effectively at the breast until they reach 34 to 36 weeks' gestational age. If your baby is born earlier than 35 weeks he is likely to need to be fed by another method for at least a short period.

Why is kangaroo care good for early babies?

Kangaroo care means carrying (or 'wearing') your baby next to your chest, inside your clothes, and is an alternative or addition to incubator care. Kangaroo care is like an advanced form of skin-to-skin contact, often with the baby secured on the mother's front with a stretchy wrap, so that she can hold him and still have her hands free. Photo number 11 shows a mother and baby in kangaroo care. Many NNUs encourage parents to provide kangaroo care because research shows that holding a baby this way means:

- He is less stressed.
- He has higher oxygen levels in his blood.
- He maintains his temperature better.
- He grows better.
- Bonding between the baby and his parents is better.
- His mother's breastmilk production is stimulated.

If the NNU staff don't suggest kangaroo care, don't be afraid to ask about it. The more you can hold your baby like this, the better.

Feeding by tube

Babies who are too weak to suck and swallow usually have their first milk feeds via a tube passed into their stomach through either their mouth or their nose. Neonatal unit staff are usually happy to show parents how to tube feed their babies – do ask if no one suggests it to you. If possible, let your baby have his feed while you are holding him against your chest, so that he can smell you and feel your skin.

WHY MIGHT A DUMMY BE RECOMMENDED?

Dummies are often used to help stimulate digestion when a baby is being tube fed. They are also used as a way of soothing a baby who is undergoing a painful procedure, or whose parents aren't available to comfort him. Dummy-sucking is sometimes referred to as non-nutritive sucking. Dummies do have a place in the care of premature babies but they can interfere with breastfeeding if they are over-used (see pages 39 and 75). Try to make sure that your baby is not given a dummy, or left sucking on one, unnecessarily.

Feeding with a dropper

Babies whose suck is weak may be able to get all the milk they need if they have small amounts put into their mouths, either expressed directly from their mother's breast or using a dropper or syringe.

Cup feeding

Babies can lap milk from an open cup before their sucking reflex develops. Many NNUs use cup feeding for babies who don't need to be tube fed but who aren't quite ready to breastfeed. Cup feeding (see page 152) is thought to be a helpful method for premature or sick babies who are going to breastfeed later because it happens at the baby's pace. Ask the staff caring for your premature baby whether he can be cup fed, and whether they can show you how to do it.

Bottle feeding

Bottle feeding is the most demanding way for a premature baby to get food. Although the milk can be made to flow readily (so sucking hard isn't necessary), the baby still needs to stop and start the flow to enable him to co-ordinate breathing and swallowing. Bottle feeding is particularly unhelpful for a baby who is going to be breastfed later, because it teaches him to expect something to be poked into his mouth, which is likely to interfere with his instinct to scoop up the breast. If you *do* need to give your baby a bottle feed, see page 151 for some tips on how to minimise the possible disruption to breastfeeding.

Helping your baby to move on to breastfeeding

As your baby matures he'll gradually move towards breast-feeding, but it's best not to rush him. As you spend time holding him skin to skin you'll notice him start to nuzzle and lick your breast and before long he'll begin to be able to move his head and arms, which will help him to find your nipple. Expressing a few drops of milk will encourage him to search for food. It's best to avoid using perfume or scented toiletries, or even washing your breasts before offering a feed, so that he learns to recognise your natural smell.

If you focus on holding your baby skin to skin so he can breastfeed as soon as he wants to, there'll be no need for anyone to decide when he is ready for his first attempt at feeding – he'll show you by doing it.

The days and weeks before your baby begins feeding at your breast are ideal for experimenting with a few different feeding positions, to help you become confident holding him in more than one way. Premature babies often have weak muscles, so they need good support for their upper back and neck. Aim to hold your baby securely, with most of his body touching you. If you're in a lying-back position with him on top of you (see page 43), all you'll need to do is steady him so he doesn't flop sideways. Upright and underarm positions can work well but be sure not to prevent your baby from tilting his head back – just like a baby born at term, he needs to be able to do this if he's to open his mouth wide and scoop up your breast at the right angle (see page 36). (See page 262 for more information on how to help babies with low muscle tone to breastfeed.)

Once your baby is showing signs of being able to feed, it's a good idea to encourage your let-down reflex before he attaches so that he won't have to make too much effort to get milk. As with a full-term baby, it's important to make sure he is effectively attached at the breast, so he can feed efficiently and give your breasts the right message. Stroking his face, especially downwards over his nose and lips, will encourage him to open his mouth and root for your breast. Nipple shields are sometimes advised for premature babies but using a shield is unlikely to help your baby to attach effectively – see page 40 for why.

Most women find that one breast has a slightly faster milk flow than the other. Offering your baby this breast first at each feed is another good way of making sure he gets milk

Breast compression can help your baby to get more milk

Breast compression is a way of increasing the flow of milk so that a baby who doesn't have much energy to feed gets plenty of milk. If, part-way into a feed, your baby is making sucking movements but has stopped swallowing, support your breast in your hand and gently close your hand around it. Apply gentle, even pressure to compress or squeeze the breast. You should notice your baby starting to swallow again. Relax your hand until he stops swallowing and then repeat the process. Be careful to use your whole hand and to avoid squeezing for longer than about a minute at a time. (If you pinch with your fingers or keep the pressure up for too long you could stop some parts of the breast from draining properly.)

quickly with the minimum of effort. If your milk flows slowly, some gentle breast compression (see above) may help to speed things up – but don't overdo it. Your baby needs time to breathe in between swallows. If you have a very fast flow or are making more milk than your baby needs, expressing some milk before he starts to feed will make the flow more gentle.

Premature babies aren't normally able to ask for feeds, so feeding them only on demand would be dangerous – they simply wouldn't get enough milk. In a neonatal unit they are usually fed on a schedule that starts with hourly feeds, then moves to two-hourly, then three-hourly. (Some NNUs may still aim for four-hour gaps, which is not realistic or helpful for breastfeeding babies.) However, once your baby gets near the age when he should have been born, he may suddenly ask for a feed before his scheduled feed is due. If you're not expecting this, it's easy to assume that breastfeeding is going wrong. In fact, he's just showing you that he's ready to regulate his own feeds, in the way that full-term babies do.

Once your baby starts asking for feeds earlier than scheduled, it's time to relax the schedule and be led by him. Provided he asks for at least eight feeds in 24 hours (or as advised by the NNU staff), you can trust him if he chooses a longer gap occasionally. You'll know he's getting enough by his general behaviour and his wees and poos (see page 97). Before long you'll be able to relax completely, allowing him to find a pattern that ensures you carry on producing the amount of milk he needs.

Breastfeeding twins (or more)

Being a parent to twins or triplets can be hugely demanding and time-consuming, especially in the early months. Most of the practical aspects of mothering take at least twice as long when there is more than one baby. But, while the practicalities of breastfeeding may take a bit of working out in the beginning, once you get going it's much less effort than making up formula feeds. It's also an ideal way to help you to bond with each of your babies.

The majority of mothers can easily produce enough milk for two or even three babies, and possibly more. And despite what friends or relatives may assume, making all this milk puts no extra physical strain on the mother. Her breasts are made for the task and **if there is twice the demand, there will be twice the supply**. Breastfeeding also makes it easy to hold and feed two babies at the same time, if that is what the mother wants to do.

However, it's common for multiple births to have the added complications of prematurity and/or Caesarean section, both of which can make it more difficult to get breastfeeding up and running (see above, and pages 64 and 63), so you are likely to need extra support from your partner or family. There are several organisations that offer specific support with the challenges of looking after more than one baby – see *Sources of information and support*, page 278, for details.

> 'Most people think breastfeeding twins will be the hardest thing in the world – but honestly, once you get going, it's the easiest option. I just can't imagine making up double lots of formula and sterilising all those bottles!'
>
> *Sarah, mother of Alex, four years, Holly and Jessica, two years*

Why bottle feeds won't make things easier

Like all breastfeeding mothers, those who have more than one baby need someone to help them with their other responsibilities while they get to grips with feeding (see Chapter 5). Making milk isn't tiring but keeping up with changing nappies, washing and dressing can be, and it's easy for those tasks to get in the way of breastfeeding.

It's common for partners or relatives to want to help mothers of multiples by offering to take over some of the feeding with a bottle. However, just as with single babies, if this happens early on it can make things harder in the long run. While giving the occasional bottle feed may seem like a kindness, it's likely, in the early weeks, to interfere with the babies' learning, making effective breastfeeding harder for them. And giving them formula will reduce the amount of milk their mother produces.

If you want to combine formula and breastfeeds, so that the feeding can be shared, it's important to allow each baby time to get the hang of breastfeeding before you introduce a bottle. This will give your babies the best chance of being able to breastfeed as well as bottle feed and will help to ensure that your breasts get a clear message, from the beginning, that they need to make plenty of milk. That way you'll be able to do as much or as little breastfeeding as you choose later on.

Mothers who are feeding more than one baby often find that their appetite is much larger than usual, but taking care of their own needs can sometimes be pushed down the list of priorities. Although not eating and drinking won't affect your milk supply, it may make you tired and irritable. Eating well and having a healthy snack and a drink every time you breastfeed is a good way to make sure you stay on top of things – so preparing meals and snacks for you is one of the best ways those around you can support you to breastfeed.

How do I feed two babies?

Holding one baby for feeding takes a bit of practice; holding two is trickier again. However, there is no need to feel you have to rush to feed two babies together. Feeding them separately can give you a chance to get to know them as individuals and to find out what works best for each one. All babies are unique and it's quite common for different feeding positions to work for each baby, and for them to feed at different speeds.

If you want to feed two babies together, lots of positions are possible. There's no need to hold both babies the same way but you do need to make sure they are close enough to your body to tilt their heads back easily to scoop up the breast, especially while you are all learning. In the early weeks a lying-back position (see page 43), with your babies on their tummies on top of you will probably be the easiest. This way they will have freedom to wriggle around to position themselves and you'll have both arms free to steady them if they need it.

Whatever feeding positions you choose, you'll probably find it helpful to have someone with you to hand over the second baby once the first has started feeding. It's a good idea to start with the baby who needs the most support to latch on (if there's a noticeable difference) so you can use both arms to help him if you need to. **Once your babies have got the hang of feeding, managing both together will be easier.**

When you are caring for two or more babies, it can feel as though you get no time to do anything else between feeds. Trying to synchronise when your babies feed can help. Breastfed babies will almost always take up an opportunity to feed if it's offered (even if they are sleepy), so unless their feeding patterns or needs are very different, you can offer both babies a feed whenever one asks, waking the second either at the same time or immediately afterwards. (It doesn't matter if one baby feeds from both breasts and the next one feeds immediately afterwards – your breasts work their hardest when they're well drained, so there's always milk available.) This strategy is definitely recommended if you are feeding more than two babies.

Sometimes mothers of twins find that one baby naturally seems to prefer the right breast and the other the left. If they are both feeding enthusiastically and effectively there is no reason to try to persuade them to swap sides. However, if one baby is noticeably weaker than the other, swapping sides can be a good idea. Allowing the stronger baby to put in the order for more milk on his twin's behalf – either at alternate feeds, or at every feed for a day or two – will mean that both breasts get the same message. It will also mean that the weaker baby doesn't have to work as hard for his food. It's particularly important to use both breasts equally for feeding and expressing if you are breastfeeding one baby but are having to express milk for the other, as sometimes happens when babies are born early.

'The twins were different at the breast. I had very fast flow on my right boob, so Jemima usually had that one because she was bigger. Harriet couldn't handle it, so she had the left breast, which had more normal flow. And they were different to get started too; Jemima always latched on really well but Harriet took ages.'

Sam, mother of George, four years, Jemima and Harriet, two years

Key points

- Breastmilk is especially important for babies who are born prematurely – and their own mother's milk is most valuable of all.

- Expressing intensively in the first two weeks is the key to meeting your premature baby's needs long term.

- Skin contact and kangaroo care help premature babies to thrive and encourage milk production. They also allow the baby to show when he is ready to move on to breastfeeding.

- Careful choices of feeding methods can help smooth the transition to breastfeeding for premature babies.

- Most mothers can produce enough milk for two, three, and even more babies. More demand = more supply.

- If you are planning to combine bottles and breast, wait until your babies have got the hang of breastfeeding before you introduce a bottle.

- Multiples often have a preference for one breast or feeding position, and feed at different speeds.

- Encouraging your babies to feed at roughly the same times will reduce the amount of time you spend feeding.

- Swapping sides is a good idea if one baby is weaker than the other(s). This ensures both breasts are told to produce plenty of milk.

12
Your milk supply

Baby-led breastfeeding makes managing your supply straight-forward. Understanding what controls how much milk you make, and the part your baby can play in changing that, is the secret to avoiding and overcoming common milk supply problems. It's even possible to start breastfeeding several weeks after your baby's birth, to go back to it after a break, or to breastfeed an adopted baby. This chapter looks at how to manage your milk production to meet common and less common challenges, as well as ways to reduce your milk supply safely if you have to stop breastfeeding early.

How milk production is determined

The number of milk-producing cells women have varies enormously (see box, below) but how rapidly an individual mother makes milk at any particular time depends on how many of her cells are up and running and how hard they are working (see Chapter 2). The number of *functioning* cells is determined in the first few weeks of breastfeeding. The more Frequent, Effective, Exclusive, on Demand and Skin to skin the feeding is (see page 71), the more cells will be primed and the greater the amount of milk the mother will be able to make for her baby (the system is reset with each pregnancy). Cells that have been primed can step their rate of production up or down, working more or less hard according to how much they are 'told' to make. This is what determines how much milk the mother is actually making at any one time.

Your capacity to produce milk is individual to you but babies are individuals, too. They have different needs and feed at different rates, so a new baby may not follow the same pattern as your last one. All of this means that each mother and baby relationship is unique when it comes to making milk.

Most mothers can make plenty of milk

Many breastfeeding mothers worry about how much milk they are producing. Often, these concerns stem from their babies' behaviour, which may be unconnected with feeding. **It's extremely rare for a mother not to be able to make enough milk to feed her baby – and there is almost always a medical problem that accounts for it** (see page 211). Yet many mothers stop breastfeeding unnecessarily in the early months because they believe they can't make enough milk.

Your capacity for milk production

Almost all women can produce enough breastmilk for at least two babies. The number of milk-producing cells each woman varies – and it has nothing to do with the size of her breasts. Some women naturally have only a small number of milk-producing cells, so each cell needs to work fairly hard most of the time. These mothers need to feed their babies very frequently to keep their milk production going at an adequate level. Other women naturally have lots of milk-making cells and struggle to keep their supply *down*. They can break all the breastfeeding rules (by feeding by the clock, using dummies, and so on) and still maintain a good level of production. Most mothers are somewhere in the middle.

Top-ups don't help

If you think you may not be producing enough milk, don't be tempted to give your baby 'top-ups' of formula. These will fill her up so that she takes less breastmilk, with the result that your milk production slows down even more.

Many common concerns, such as an unsettled baby, frequent feeding, wakefulness at night, slow weight gain and only being able to express small amounts, are assumed to indicate a lack of milk but none of these is a reliable sign that the baby isn't getting enough. For example, wanting to feed frequently is normal for a breastfed baby, while unsettled behaviour and crying can have many different causes. Even if the baby is currently not getting all the milk she needs, this doesn't mean her mother isn't capable of producing enough.

'I think you always worry that you won't have enough milk but if they're happy and putting on weight, it must be okay.'

Gina, mother of Micah, four months

Almost all mothers produce plenty of milk for their baby in the first week or so but this doesn't carry on if the milk isn't removed effectively and frequently. If your baby is not spending enough time at the breast, or not feeding efficiently when she is there (or both), your breasts will soon stop producing the milk she needs. This doesn't mean your milk supply is running out or drying up – just that your baby hasn't been putting in a big enough order.

Provided your milk production was 'kick-started' with lots of effective feeding (or expressing) in the first few days (see Chapters 5 and 11), the capacity for you to make lots of milk is always present – you just need to tell your breasts that

NOT ENOUGH MILK – A WESTERN PROBLEM

In communities where it's usual for babies to be carried next to their mother's breast all day, a baby will help herself to a few sucks every 20 to 30 minutes. Not having enough milk is almost unknown in these societies. In the UK, most babies have to ask for feeds, so they tend to feed much less frequently than this. For many women, feeding their baby fewer than eight to ten times a day means they will struggle to meet her needs.

more is wanted. However, if you didn't get the chance to breastfeed or express your milk in the first few days there may be a limit to how much you can increase production (see page 23). It's still important, though, to help your breasts to start making more milk than they have been, by increasing the stimulation you give them now.

If you think your baby isn't getting enough milk

If you suspect that your baby may not be getting enough milk, start by checking the signs that breastfeeding is working. As explained in Chapter 6, her wees and poos will provide the best clues (as long as she is having only breast-milk – no water, formula or other food), followed by her behaviour and weight. There are four likely scenarios:

1) **If your baby is weeing and pooing normally for her age and is gaining weight** it's unlikely that she isn't getting enough milk. If she just seems to be feeding very frequently (and has always done so), this is probably her natural pattern. If she's unsettled and needing to feed more frequently than usual, maybe:

- she's going through an appetite (or 'growth') spurt (see page 112)
- she's teething, or coming down with a cold
- she's feeling the need for extra comfort (is there anything going on in the household that could be unsettling her?)
- her natural feeding pattern is changing as she grows older.

2) **If your baby is weeing and pooing normally but *not* gaining weight,** this suggests she *is* getting enough milk but that she has another health problem. It would be advisable to get her checked by your doctor.

3) **If your baby is producing lots of watery, green poo and is very miserable (or 'colicky')** she may be getting the wrong balance of sugar and fat in her feed. See page 102 for how to remedy this.

4) **If your baby is not producing normal amounts of wee and poo (and isn't gaining weight) but seems otherwise well,** the most likely problem is that she *isn't* getting enough milk. See below for what to do to improve her intake.

If your baby isn't getting enough milk, it's probably related to the way she's feeding. For a baby under two weeks old, adjusting the attachment may be all that's needed but, if there's still a problem, it's likely to be that she's either not feeding often enough or is coming off the breast too early. If in doubt, remember, more **FEEDS** = more milk (see page 71). If your baby is older than two weeks, it's likely that your milk production will have started to slow down, so the problem may take a bit longer to resolve. Either way, here's how to help her get more milk:

- *Check your baby's attachment at the breast* (see page 50). **This is the first thing to do, because the rest won't work if she isn't able to feed effectively.** Is her chin indenting your breast? Is her mouth open wide and are her cheeks full? Can you see or hear her swallowing frequently? If not, you may need to hold her in a slightly different way so that she can tilt her head back more or come to the breast at a different angle.

- Unless there are serious medical concerns about her wellbeing, **don't give your baby anything else to eat or drink other than your breastmilk.** Your breasts need to be told what her true needs are.

- *Watch for your baby's subtle feeding cues* (see page 75) – are you missing any signals that she might want to feed?

- *Encourage your baby to feed more often.* If she's sleepy and doesn't seem interested, try expressing a few drops of milk on to her lips to tempt her. Holding her skin to skin may help to awaken her instincts.

- *Make sure your baby is close to you at night,* so you can feed her as soon as she stirs.

- *Avoid using a dummy,* which could stop your baby (and you) realising that she needs to feed.

- If you've previously been taking her off the breast when you think she's had enough, **let your baby feed for as long as she wants on each breast.** If she's feeding effectively she *will* let go when she's had what she needs.

- *Always offer your baby the second breast* (but don't worry if she doesn't want it).

In most cases, more frequent feeding (with effective attachment) is all that's needed to enable a baby to get more milk. However, if breastfeeding has not been going well for more than a week, your milk production may have slowed down significantly. In this case the best way to turn things around is to give your breasts a wake-up call by following a plan of intensive feeding or expressing (or a combination of both). The next section explains how to do this.

Giving your supply an intensive boost

This concentrated feeding plan should quickly get your breasts working hard, and producing lots more milk. You'll need to do this if you think your milk production has been low for more than a week. It's a mini version of the baby-moon described in Chapter 5. Here's how it works:

- If possible, arrange for someone else to be around to take on your usual responsibilities so that you can focus on breastfeeding.
- Find somewhere safe, warm and comfortable where you can stay in skin-to-skin contact with your baby while you are awake (your bed, or the sofa, for example). This is your 'nest'.
- Keep plenty of drinks and snacks within arm's reach, so you don't have to keep getting up.
- Stay in your 'nest' as much as you can and encourage your baby to have *lots* of breastfeeds – *at least* one every two hours but more often if she's willing. It doesn't matter if they are very short – the more often she feeds, the more your breasts will be stimulated to make milk.
- If you can't encourage your baby to feed at least every two hours, try switch feeding at each feed (see box, above) and express your milk in between feeds.
- Continue to feed your baby as often as you can throughout the night.

If your baby isn't keen to feed frequently, expressing between feeds will make sure that your breasts are given a big enough order to make more milk. However, this won't work if you give your baby the milk you have expressed every time, because then she won't go to the breast as often as she otherwise would – so your breasts will take longer to get the

---

Helping a sleepy baby to get more milk

'Switch feeding' is a short-term measure that can help a baby who tires quickly to get more milk. If your baby falls asleep after only a few minutes of feeding, swapping her to the other side will wake her up a bit and encourage her to start feeding again. It will also trigger a new let-down reflex, which will help her to get more milk without too much effort. If she falls asleep again, switch her back to the first breast. Feed by feed, if she is effectively attached, she'll start to feed for longer on each side and you'll find yourself having to switch her less often. Within a few days, you'll be able to stop switching altogether.

REMEDIES THAT *MAY* HELP YOU MAKE MORE MILK

Galactogogues are medicines and herbal remedies that can help boost milk production. Some mothers find them helpful but they don't replace the need to feed or express frequently. In the past, mothers whose babies were in a neonatal unit were often prescribed domperidone or metoclopramide to increase their milk supply. However, recent evidence suggests that the sort of intensive boost described above is much more likely to bring about a significant and lasting increase in milk supply than taking medications. If you *do* decide to take medicines or herbs, make sure they are prescribed by a registered practitioner.

message. It's best to save any breastmilk you express and give it to your baby only if she is unsettled and offering her the breast doesn't calm her. (If you have already started giving her some formula feeds, see page 220 for how to phase these out as your milk supply improves.)

How can I tell that I'm making more milk?

As always, your baby's wees and poos are the best guide to how much milk she's getting (see page 97) – more out means there must be more going in. As she begins to take more milk her behaviour will change, too. If she was unsettled and crying, she will start to be happier and may ask for feeds less often. However, if she was a very quiet, sleepy baby, she will probably start to be more wakeful and keen to feed.

If your baby is under two weeks old and her attachment at the breast was the main cause of the problem, you will probably find that your breasts now feel noticeably less full after feeds. If she's older, and your milk production had gone down, you may begin to feel full before feeds again.

If you don't start to see changes in your baby's behaviour and an improvement in her wees and poos within 48 hours, seek help from someone skilled in helping with breastfeeding (see *Where can I get help?*, page 106).

Less common reasons for low milk production

Although low milk production can usually be fixed with minor adjustments to the way you feed, there are some other possible causes. The first two are the most likely culprits:

- The contraceptive pill (especially the combined pill), contraceptive implants and hormone-based coils (IUSs) can interfere with your hormone balance and reduce milk production. Tell your doctor or family planning nurse that you are breastfeeding before you decide to use one of these methods.

- The presence of small pieces of the placenta that have been left behind in the womb (known as retained products of conception) can trick your body into thinking you are still pregnant. If your tummy is tender, if you are passing fresh blood more than four days after the birth or if you have a smelly vaginal discharge, contact your midwife or doctor as soon as possible.

- Some common medicines can be a problem. Decongestants can decrease milk production and anti-histamines can make a baby drowsy and cause her to ask for fewer feeds. If you need to take medication, check that it won't affect your milk production (see pages 133 and 255).

- Smoking and drinking alcohol have been shown to have a *small* effect on the amount of available milk but this is negligible if feeding is baby-led.

- Some babies who are premature or have physical problems may need help to feed effectively (see Chapters 11 and 15).

- A very few women have a condition that may reduce their ability to produce breastmilk, for example polycystic ovary syndrome or an underactive thyroid gland.

Could I be making too much milk?

Although it's a less common concern than not having enough milk, women who produce too much milk can find breast-feeding problematic. If you are producing more milk than your baby needs, your breasts will probably be uncomfortable for much of the time. They are likely to leak a lot, and, if they are very heavy, they may cause backache. The flow of milk may make your baby feel as though she is drowning during feeds. She may clamp her jaws together or pull away to try to stop the flow, or come off the breast coughing and spluttering. She may also show signs of colic (see page 102). It's easy for mothers (and their families) to interpret this behaviour as being due to not enough milk, or milk that isn't strong enough to satisfy the baby, but this is not the case.

Am I really making too much?

If you suspect that you are producing too much milk, it's important to make sure this is true before doing anything to tackle it. Many of the signs mentioned above can have other causes. For example, during the first few weeks it's normal for mothers to make more milk than their baby needs and for babies to struggle with the rush of milk at the beginning of a feed. And because this is when long-term milk production is being set up, it's important not to do anything to suppress milk production during this time.

Even after the first few weeks, other causes for what appears to be too much milk are possible: breasts can feel overfull because they are not being drained effectively; some mothers have a very strong let-down reflex or readily leak milk, even though they are producing normal amounts; a baby can show 'colicky' behaviour for all sorts of reasons, including not being effectively attached at the breast; and some babies with muscular or neurological problems (see Chapter 15) have difficulty coping with even a relatively gentle flow of milk.

To be sure that the likely cause of the problems you are experiencing is that you are producing too much milk, check the following:

- Your baby was not born before 37 weeks of pregnancy.
- She is over three weeks old.
- She is well and developing normally.

- She is gaining weight well (or very fast).
- She is unsettled most of the time, and asking to feed very frequently.
- She is passing lots of urine and watery, green stools.
- She always attaches effectively at the breast (see page 50).
- Your breasts feel full most of the time.

If any of these *don't* apply, or you are unsure whether your baby is attaching effectively at the breast, speak to someone skilled in helping with breastfeeding (see *Where can I get help?*, page 106) before doing anything to reduce milk production. If you are in any doubt about your baby's general health and development, see your doctor or health visitor first.

'I always had a lot of milk – I'd have to change my breast pads every time I changed a nappy and I was always leaking. I just thought it was normal. As soon as he latched on, Alfie used to pull away spluttering and milk would squirt all over him. At 10 weeks he started getting green watery poos that "fizzed" and every evening he'd have terrible colic. And he was hungry all the time. It settled down a bit when he was about six months, and it wasn't until after that – when I was looking through a breastfeeding book for something else – that I realised I'd had over-supply. I had no idea there was anything I could have done.'

Sara, mother of Alfie, five years

What to do if you're making too much milk

A mother who isn't producing enough milk can feed her baby more frequently to increase her supply, but as someone who is inclined to make too much milk you can't just cut down the number of feeds your baby has. Your milk is digested as fast as any other mother's and your baby's stomach can only hold so much at one time, so she will still need to feed fairly frequently. But that doesn't mean there's nothing you can do to make things easier for you both.

Mothers who have a tendency to overproduce can easily get into a vicious cycle that works like this:

- The mother produces more milk than her baby can manage at a feed.
- The baby feeds well but gets full up before she reaches the creamiest milk.
- She is hungry again very soon because she didn't get many calories.
- Her mother's breasts get over-stimulated by the frequent feeding and *increase* milk production.
- The baby gets full up even earlier at each feed. She is 'colicky' – and both she and her mother are miserable.

Most babies of mothers who are making too much milk don't need both breasts every time they feed, and letting your baby feed from just one side may be all that's needed. If the other breast feels uncomfortable, express some milk – just enough to relieve the discomfort. Leaving milk in the breasts helps to slow down production (see page 25), so after a day or two you may not need to express. Using each breast only half as often may be enough to keep your milk production at a reasonable level.

If your baby is having only one breast each time she feeds and you still have a problem, the answer may be to express a small amount of milk beforehand, so that she doesn't have to wade through so much low-fat milk before she gets to the creamier stuff. That way she'll get a smaller, higher-calorie feed, which will cure her tummy-ache and stop her needing to feed again quite so soon. Less frequent feeding will gradually encourage your breasts to slow down production. You'll need to use trial and error to work out how much to express – start with just a few teaspoonfuls and see if that's enough to make your baby happier. When your breasts start to feel less full between feeds you can try feeding without expressing first, to see if your strategy has worked. Many women who overproduce find that expressing a little before each feed for a day or two every few weeks is enough to keep the problem under control.

The 'clearout' method is a more radical solution. This involves expressing as much milk as you can from both breasts in one go. Then, at your baby's next feed, you offer her just one breast – and keep offering that one whenever she wants to feed during the next three to four hours. (If she comes off that side and seems to want more you can offer her the other one, but it's unlikely this will happen if your over-production is extreme.) Then you switch to the other breast and restrict her to that one for the next few hours.

This approach may seem strange (and it isn't exactly baby-led) but it works by 'resting' each breast in turn, which stops them from constantly topping themselves up. And, because they start fully drained, engorgement is unlikely. Many mothers who've used the clearout method find they can go back to a normal breastfeeding pattern after four or five days. Others find they need to stick to a one-side-for-three-hours rule indefi-nitely. Usually, though, the clearout doesn't need to be repeated.

REMEDIES TO SLOW DOWN MILK PRODUCTION

Anti-galactogogues are medicines and herbal remedies that can help reduce milk production. If your overproduction isn't controllable by the methods described above you may want to consult a doctor, herbalist or lactation consultant to see if they can suggest something that will help. (As with any other medications, make sure they are prescribed by a registered practitioner and that it's safe for your baby to have your milk while you're taking them.)

Starting breastfeeding when you haven't just given birth

Breastfeeding usually starts soon after a baby is born but sometimes it doesn't begin until some time later. This may be because the mother didn't want to breastfeed initially but then changed her mind, or it may be that she wants to re-start after a break. Sometimes a mother wants to breastfeed her adopted baby, or one born to a surrogate mother. All of these are possible, although the level of milk production achieved varies enormously, depending on the circumstances. In each case, the individual woman's determination to make it work and the support of those around her are key factors.

If you want to start breastfeeding in one of these situations, it's a good idea to talk to a breastfeeding counsellor or lactation consultant, who will be able to help you develop a personalised plan based on the principles outlined below.

Starting breastfeeding late

It's never too late to decide to breastfeed your baby. However, the longer the gap between the birth and getting started, the lower your chances will be of reaching full milk production. If it's only been a week, the likelihood is that you'll be able to revert to breastfeeding very quickly and you may not need to follow all the steps described below. If it's longer than that, you may have to work a little harder. In some cases, full breastfeeding won't be possible but partial breastfeeding, with some formula feeds, almost certainly will. **The information in this section will also be relevant for you if things didn't go well in the early days of breastfeeding and your baby is now having formula for some or all of her feeds.**

In the first few weeks after birth, if a mother's milk-producing cells sense that milk isn't needed, they start to shut down. Once this happens, they can't be re-activated until her next pregnancy. How quickly the shut-down happens varies from mother to mother and, unfortunately, there is no way of telling, in the days and weeks after the birth, how many milk-making cells are active. The only way to find out how much milk you can make is to give it a go.

When beginning breastfeeding some time after your baby's birth, or recovering from a difficult start, you are likely to be faced with two challenges: getting your breasts into milk-making mode and persuading your baby to feed from them. If your baby is happy to latch on to your breast, she will be able to put in most of the order for milk herself. However, if she has never breastfed effectively she may take a while to figure out what to do. In that case you will need to rely mainly on expressing to get your breasts working. Once they are producing more milk, persuading your baby to latch on will be easier.

There are three main ways to get your breasts to start making milk:

- *An intensive supply boost* is the quickest and most effective method. See page 209 for how to do this.

- *Waking up your breasts gradually, over a week or two* (see below) may suit you better if you want to take things more slowly.

- *Using a breastfeeding supplementer* (see page 219) is a gradual alternative but it can be fiddly, so it's not ideal for short-term use.

Here's what to do if you want to stimulate your breasts to return to milk making over a period of a week or two:

- Offer your baby the chance to breastfeed as often as you can (don't wait until she's hungry). Hold her so she can nuzzle against your breast when she's drifting off to sleep or just stirring awake.

- Hold your baby skin to skin as much as possible. This will help her to feel safe and happy near your breast and stimulate you to release the hormones you need to make milk. If possible, carry her skin to skin in a sling so you can continue to hold her even when you need your hands free for something else.

- Hold your baby next to your breast when you're bottle feeding her. If you can, express a little breastmilk and smear a few drops over the teat before you offer her the bottle, to help her associate feeding with the smell of your breastmilk.

- When you're offering your baby a bottle feed, brush the teat down over the tip of her nose and her top lip to encourage her to tilt her head back, open her mouth wide and reach forward with her tongue – as she will need to do at the breast.

FEEDING YOUR BABY WITH A BREASTFEEDING SUPPLEMENTER

A breastfeeding (or 'nursing') supplementer is a bottle with a fine tube that it is taped to the breast so that the tip extends to the tip of the nipple. The bottle is filled with either formula or expressed breast-milk. The baby takes the tube and the breast into her mouth when she feeds, stimulating the breast to make milk while she gets milk from the tube.

A supplementer allows a baby to have feeds of expressed breast-milk or formula at the breast. It can be used to help a mother relactate (see page 221) or to start or boost milk production for a baby who isn't able to take much from her mother's breast directly. If long-term supplementation is needed, it can provide an alternative to bottles. A breastfeeding specialist will be able to discuss the pros and cons of supplementers with you, and show you how to use one.

- Massage your breasts and nipples and hand express in between feeding opportunities.

Once your baby is breastfeeding frequently, watching her behaviour at the breast (and especially her swallowing, see page 92) will give you clues as to how much milk she's getting and help you work out when to start phasing out her formula feeds.

How to phase out your baby's formula feeds

As your breasts start to produce milk and you can see your baby swallowing during feeds you will be able to start reducing the amount of formula she has. You can do this by giving gradually smaller amounts at each feed over a period of several days or weeks – or you can go for a more rapid changeover, like this:

- Follow the intensive supply boost on page 209, setting up your 'nest' with drinks and snacks to hand and focusing on having plenty of skin contact with your baby – and *lots* of breastfeeds (as often as every half hour, if your baby is willing).
- Offer your baby a bottle feed only when she is no longer content to feed at the breast. If possible, get someone else to give that feed so that your baby associates you solely with breastfeeding. Don't try to persuade her to finish the bottle.
- Go back to your 'nest' with your baby and continue with skin contact and lots of breastfeeding.

This approach will boost your milk production very quickly, so that breastfeeding can take over from most or all of the formula feeding within two or three days. It will also save you having to calculate how much formula to give at each feed.

Whichever method you choose, you will need to keep an eye on your baby's wees and poos, throughout, and for at least a week after you stop giving formula, just to confirm that you're producing enough breastmilk for her. Don't expect her feeding pattern to be the same as it was, though, especially if she was sleeping for a long period overnight; breastfeeding is meant to happen frequently, day and night.

If you don't seem to be able to get rid of the formula feeds completely, you've probably found your maximum milk production level. In that case, you can decide when is the most convenient time of day (or night) for your baby to have the formula she still needs, so that you can continue to breastfeed her frequently the rest of the time. (Tip: Don't assume that the obvious time to give formula is going to be at night; breastfeeding is usually quicker and simpler than preparing a bottle and will help both of you get back to sleep quickly – see page 113.)

Can I produce milk after a break from breastfeeding?

Sometimes mothers who have breastfed their baby in the past want to start again after a break. This is known as relactation. In some countries, it's not unusual for a grandmother to relactate so she can help feed her grandchild. In the UK, it tends to happen when a mother who stopped breastfeeding after a few weeks changes her mind. If the period of breastfeeding was very brief or difficult, the situation will be more similar to starting breastfeeding late and you can relactate using any one of the three possible approaches described on page 220.

Restarting milk production is easier the shorter the gap since breastfeeding stopped – but it's never too late. It just takes more commitment the longer you've left it.

Can I breastfeed an adopted baby?

It is possible to breastfeed an adopted baby (or your own biological baby, born to a surrogate mother) but how easy you will find it, and how much milk you will be able to make, depends on your breastfeeding history, on how old the baby is when you take over her care, and on whether she has breastfed before.

If you have previously fully breastfed one or more babies, even if it was a long time ago, you will in effect be relactating, so your chances of achieving full milk production will be quite high. However, if you haven't breastfed before – and especially if you've never been pregnant – then you will be inducing lactation rather than reactivating it. In this case full breastfeeding may not be possible.

It may be that your main aim in choosing to breastfeed is to provide your baby with your breastmilk, perhaps for specific health reasons. Or it may be that what you want most is to be able to nurture her at your breast, because of the emotional closeness this will bring. Your best course of action depends on which of these matters most to you.

If you are keen to produce as much breastmilk as you can, then – ideally – you will need to start stimulating your breasts to produce milk several months in advance. Some specific methods for inducing lactation have been developed, which include a prescribed course of hormones, followed by a combination of drugs or herbal medicines and intensive breast stimulation and expression. If you want to follow this sort of protocol, we suggest you contact a lactation consultant (see *Sources of information and support*, page 278). If you don't want to go to these lengths, you can do an extended version of the two-week 'wake-up call' described on page 189, instead. Expect it to take a couple of weeks for milk to start to appear, and several more for production to build up.

If feeding your baby at your breast is more important to you than producing breastmilk, then you may prefer simply to have lots of skin contact with her, and give her formula feeds via a breastfeeding supplementer (see page 219).

If you are lucky, your adopted baby will have been breast-fed at some time in the past – possibly even right up until the adoption. However, it's more likely she will be used to bottle feeding, in which case see page 126 and page 219 for some suggestions that will help her to be happy feeding at the breast. In the case of a surrogacy arrangement, you may be able to hold your baby skin to skin as soon as she's born (see page 55), in which case persuading her to accept your breast is unlikely to be a problem.

If you need (or want) to stop breastfeeding early

This section is about stopping breastfeeding completely while your baby is under a year old and still reliant on breastmilk. For information about ending breastfeeding when your baby is older, see page 176. For information about stopping breast-feeding temporarily (for example, for medical reasons), see page 145.

If you have decided you need, or want, to stop breastfeed-ing completely, and your baby is under a year old, you'll need to help her make the transition to formula feeds (see below). You will also need to consider how to manage your own comfort.

Stopping breastfeeding is best done gradually, for the sake of both you and your baby. If you do it suddenly your breasts won't immediately recognise what has happened, so for a while they will carry on producing milk at their previ-ous rate. If you don't remove at least some of this milk you risk, at best, the discomfort of overfull breasts or, at worst, mastitis.

You can help your breasts to wind down production slowly by cutting down your baby's breastfeeds step by step, or more quickly by expressing your milk. Either way, you can expect milk production to take several weeks to stop completely.

How to stop breastfeeding gradually

The gentlest way to switch from breastfeeding to formula feeding is as follows:

- Start by working out the average pattern of your baby's main breastfeeds over each 24-hour period.
- Replace one of these breastfeeds with a formula feed.
- Allow your breasts two or three days to adjust their rate of milk production before dropping the next breastfeed. Repeat this until all breastfeeds have been replaced.
- Try to avoid eliminating consecutive breastfeeds one after the other. Instead, alternate between feeds at opposite times of the day (or night), so that the gaps between the remaining breastfeeds stay more or less even.
- Aim to leave the times that your baby most enjoys feeding (commonly first thing in the morning and evenings or night times) till last.
- Replace occasional, very brief feeds with a drink, snack, cuddle or distracting activity.
- If you get uncomfortably full between breastfeeds, express a little milk to soften your breasts slightly. This will help prevent you becoming engorged and make it easier for your baby to attach when she next goes to the breast.

How to stop breastfeeding quickly

To end breastfeeding quickly, simply replace all your baby's breastfeeds with formula and express your milk instead. There is no need to express very much milk at a time – just do it as often and for as long as you need to remain comfortable.

Using your comfort as a guide is the best way to avoid engorgement. If you save the milk you express (see *How to store breastmilk*, page 149), you can give it to your baby occasionally in place of a formula feed.

After a few days you'll probably find that you need to express only two or three times a day, and this will be down to once a day after a week or so. However, although spontaneous leaking and fullness will disappear quite quickly, don't expect to get to a point where you can't express any milk at all. The breasts are meant to make milk, not to absorb it, and it's not unusual for mothers to be able to express milk many months (or even years) after they last breastfed.

Bottles don't have the same built-in comfort factor as breastfeeding, so be sure to hold your baby close while you give her formula feeds. You may find that she benefits from extra cuddles and from some skin contact. (This may work better with another family member at first, so that she is not frustrated by the smell of your breastmilk.)

Whether you choose a gradual changeover to formula or a rapid one, you may decide that you are happy, after all, to keep one or two breastfeeds a day (or more), rather than stopping entirely. In that case your breasts will simply settle to producing the amount of milk those feeds require. You will find things work best (and that your breasts are most comfortable) if the remaining breastfeeds are evenly spaced throughout the day – for example, at bedtime and first thing in the morning. And, of course, if you change your mind completely, you can reverse the down-scaling of your milk production just by breastfeeding more often.

Key points

- Milk production is very flexible – especially when breastfeeding has got off to a good start. It can be increased or reduced, just by changing the 'order'.

- Some women naturally produce less milk than others but almost all mothers can produce plenty of milk for their baby.

- A few women have a tendency to make too much milk but there are ways of managing this situation.

- If you opt for formula feeding when your baby is born and then decide to breastfeed, you can swap over. The sooner you do so, the more likely you are to be able to breastfeed fully.

- If you stop breastfeeding and then change your mind, you can start again.

- You may be able to produce breastmilk for an adopted baby, or one born to a surrogate mother.

- Stopping breastfeeding before one year is best done gradually – for your sake and your baby's.

13

When breastfeeding hurts

Breastfeeding isn't meant to hurt; yet many mothers stop feeding before they really want to because they are in pain. The most common painful conditions are sore nipples, engorgement, blocked ducts and mastitis. Mostly, these conditions can be avoided if breastfeeding is baby-led but they may still happen occasionally. This chapter looks at what causes breast and nipple pain and what to do to get breastfeeding back on track if it happens to you. (You may find it helpful to turn to the *Painful breastfeeding: quick symptom checker* on page 275 for an at-a-glance summary.

Is it the milk let-down?

If your baby is under a month old, the first thing to rule out if breastfeeding hurts is a painful let-down. The let-down reflex happens near the beginning of a feed when the hormone oxytocin makes the tiny muscles in the breast contract to squeeze the milk down the ducts. For most women, if this is noticed at all, it's felt as a slight tingling sensation. However, some mothers experience it as a painful pinching or squeezing inside the breast, lasting up to about 10 seconds.

A painful let-down is distinguishable from other types of breast pain because it tends to come on near the beginning of a feed (or between feeds, if something triggers it) and is accompanied by the baby swallowing more rapidly or by milk leaking. It happens in *both* breasts simultaneously and is often stronger in the breast that is not being fed from.

Most mothers who experience a painful let-down reflex find that it is only a problem in the first few weeks, while their body is adjusting to breastfeeding, and that it gradually becomes less painful. In the meantime, relaxation techniques – even those used during labour, such as slow breathing – can be useful. Humming or tapping your fingers to distract you from the pain can also help.

Sore nipples – why they happen and what to do

It's quite likely you'll experience some nipple tenderness in the early days, while you and your baby are learning how to breastfeed. But it shouldn't last for more than the first 10 seconds of each feed – and it shouldn't still be happening after the first week. If your nipples are painful for longer than a brief 'ouch' moment at the beginning of each feed in the first week (page 38), or are sore at any time after this, the pain is almost certainly caused by either injury or infection. This sort of pain won't go away by itself, so it needs to be sorted out.

Sore nipples caused by trauma or injury

A mother's nipple can be injured when her baby isn't attached to the breast effectively. If he doesn't have a big mouthful of breast, the nipple will be either squashed against the roof of his mouth (the hard palate) or subjected to excessively strong suction – or both. Nipples that are being injured during feeds usually start off just feeling sore but, if the problem isn't dealt with, the skin quickly gets damaged, leading to cracks and bleeding. Some women seem to be more prone to skin damage than others but the cause of injured nipples – ineffective attachment – is the same in every case.

A crack across the tip of the nipple is caused by the nipple being repeatedly squashed during feeding. If your nipple looks an odd shape when your baby releases it, especially if it's wedge-shaped or has a white line across it, or is blue-ish or very pale, it's probably being pinched in a way that will lead to a crack developing.

A crack or tear around the base of the nipple happens when the nipple is repeatedly sucked backwards and forwards in the baby's mouth, stretching it so that the skin gives way. This tends to happen if the baby hasn't been able to draw the nipple far enough into his mouth. If you see your breast moving in and out of your baby's mouth while he's feeding, this sort of damage is likely to happen.

If a mother doesn't hold her baby close enough for him to be able to scoop up the breast and draw the nipple deeply into his mouth, it's easy for the nipple to be injured. A vicious cycle can develop if it has already been damaged and feeding is painful, making the mother too frightened of the pain to bring her baby in close enough, and leading to further damage.

Damaged nipples are a sign that your baby isn't feeding effectively – which means he won't be getting as much milk from your breast as he should. As well as being a problem for both of you *now*, ineffective feeding can soon start to affect how much milk you are producing, so it's important not to ignore it.

Occasionally, nipple damage is caused by a tongue tie (see page 40). This can be remedied fairly easily if it's diagnosed early and the baby referred to a specialist.

Treating injured nipples

If one or both of your nipples are cracked you need to help your baby to improve his attachment to the breast urgently – with expert help if necessary. Unless they are infected (see below) your nipples won't require treatment – once they are no longer being damaged at every feed, the cracks will heal within a day or two – but if you carry on feeding as you have been in spite of the pain, the damage will get worse.

Although it may seem logical to 'rest' a damaged nipple to allow it to heal, this will only work in the short term. If your baby's attachment isn't improved, your nipple will almost certainly get sore again as soon as he goes back to feeding from it. On the other hand, **once the attachment is 'right' you should find it's possible to feed without pain, even from a nipple that is badly damaged, while allowing it to begin to heal at the same time.** If you can't get help quickly to change the way your baby is feeding, and feel it's too painful to carry on, you'll need to express your milk (from one or both breasts, depending how sore they are) so that you don't become engorged. This will also allow your baby to continue having only your milk. But improving his attachment should be your priority.

To help your baby to attach well, you'll probably need to experiment with different ways to hold him. There's a list of signs to watch for on page 50. Ask your partner, mother, sister or a close friend to watch him feed – or watch him yourself, in a mirror. Bear in mind that different things work for different mothers and babies, so what works for a friend may not work for you.

While you are helping your baby to attach more effectively, you may want to offer him the less painful breast first at each feed, so that he is not as hungry when he feeds from the more painful side. If you're not sure how effective your baby's attachment is, or you are still in pain even though he appears to be feeding well, contact someone who is skilled at helping with breastfeeding (see *Where can I get help?*, page 106).

'I found the first few weeks of breastfeeding very hard. We had lots of visitors over the first few days, and one day my nipple started to bleed as I was feeding. My friend said: "Don't worry, that always happens – it won't do the baby any harm." So I didn't ask for help for ages. By the time I talked to a breastfeeding supporter my nipple was so badly cracked I'd got to the point where I was scared to feed because of the pain.'

Gemma, mother of Jack, eight months

Most products on the market (especially nipple creams) that claim to prevent or treat sore and cracked nipples don't actually do either, although they may make sore nipples feel a little more comfortable. If you have a very sore nipple, applying a little breastmilk will do a similar job and will also help to prevent infection. When you are at home, going topless will prevent friction from clothes.

I'VE GOT BLOOD IN MY MILK!

Sometimes a baby will bring up milk which has blood in it. There's no need to panic if this happens to you. If the blood looks fresh it's almost certainly your blood, not your baby's. And it probably looks a lot more than it really is.

Swallowing blood is not harmful and it's unlikely that the blood made your baby sick. However, bleeding from the breast or nipple is a sign that something is wrong, so it needs attention.

The first thing to do is check your nipples for signs of injury. If there is nothing obvious and your nipples don't feel sore, the bleeding is probably the result of increased blood flow and rapid development of the milk-producing tissue (sometimes known as 'rusty pipe syndrome' – see also page 28). Alternatively, it may be coming from a skin tag (or papilloma) in one of your ducts.

Bleeding from increased blood flow or a papilloma should stop within a week or two of your baby's birth. If you have bleeding from within the breast that lasts more than a couple of weeks it's probably a good idea to have it checked by your doctor.

A cracked nipple will be more painful if the skin is allowed to dry out and a scab forms. You can prevent this by smearing a tiny amount of a plain, unscented, lanolin-based ointment or petroleum jelly over the crack after each feed. (This will also help to stop your breast pad or bra sticking to it and causing pain when you peel it off.) As long as you keep the amount small, there's no need to wash it off before your baby feeds again.

Nipple shields are sometimes suggested for sore nipples but they are best avoided because they tend to encourage the baby to feed in a way that isn't effective. They can also rub against the nipple, causing more damage.

Sore nipples caused by an infection

The two main types of nipple infection are bacterial infection and thrush (candida – a fungal infection). Both cause severe pain in the nipple itself. Some women experience referred pain deeper within the breast as well but, in general, deep breast pain is more usually caused by mastitis (see page 240).

Bacterial infection

Nipples that have been damaged can occasionally pick up a bacterial infection, although this isn't very common – mainly because they're being bathed in breastmilk several times a day, which protects them. If you do see pus around your nipple, or coming from it, you need to consult your doctor, who will probably prescribe a course of antibiotics. It will normally be safe for you to continue to feed your baby from that breast. To avoid further damage, you'll also need to work on making sure your baby's attachment is effective (see Chapter 3).

Thrush

Some women are more prone to thrush than others but the risk of contracting it is slightly higher if you are taking

Is it really thrush?

Soreness caused by ineffective attachment can easily be mistaken for thrush. Ask a breastfeeding specialist to check whether your baby is finding it difficult to attach (perhaps because you are trying to hold him in a position that he has outgrown) before you jump to the conclusion that you have thrush.

oral contraceptives or steroids, have recently had a course of antibiotics or if your baby is using a dummy.

Unless you have taken (or been given) antibiotics around the time of the birth, thrush is unlikely in the early weeks of breastfeeding. Usually, it appears 'out of the blue' after a period of problem-free feeding. It usually starts on one breast and is quickly spread by the baby to the other breast.

The main symptom of thrush is severe burning pain, which comes on during a feed and continues, or worsens, after the feed is over (unlike the pain of damaged nipples, which immediately lessens when the baby lets go). Some women describe this as being like 'bee stings' or 'feeding through broken glass'. Other possible symptoms are:

- shiny or flaky skin on or around the nipples
- skin which is more pink or red than usual
- itchiness around the nipples
- cracks in the nipples that refuse to heal, despite effective attachment.

If you have thrush your baby will probably be infected too. You may be able to see white patches inside his mouth but these aren't always visible. Some babies with thrush pull off the breast during feeds because their mouth is sore. The infection passes through the digestive system, so babies who have oral thrush often have a sore bottom as well.

Thrush doesn't mean you have to stop breastfeeding. However, you and your baby will need specific treatment. In the meantime, paracetamol or ibuprofen may help. It's a good idea to pay attention to your baby's feeding technique, too, because pain (for either of you) can interfere with attachment at the breast.

Nipple thrush can be very persistent. Treatment usually starts with an anti-fungal cream but many women find they need to take tablets as well. It's usual to need to continue the treatment for *at least* a week. (The single-dose remedies that are sold over the counter for vaginal thrush are not effective against nipple thrush.) Your baby will need his own medication (for his mouth, and possibly his bottom). Make sure your doctor provides you with separate prescriptions so that you don't keep passing the infection back to one another.

Letting your skin breathe will help to discourage thrush. Choose a cotton bra – or, better still, no bra at all. If you use breast pads, choose those without a waterproof backing and change them frequently. Avoiding yeasty and sugary foods and eating plenty of live yoghurt may also help to prevent an attack.

Thrush can survive on washable nappies, towels, bras, teats, dummies and toys. Boil whatever you can and wash the rest in hot soapy water, rinsing thoroughly. Ironing your bra can help to kill stubborn thrush spores. And make sure each member of the family has his or her own towel until the thrush has gone. To be on the safe side, it's best not to save any breastmilk expressed while you have thrush, as it could re-infect your baby if it's given to him later (even if it's been frozen).

Sometimes thrush doesn't clear up (or recurs quickly) because someone else in the family has it, without knowing. If your partner or older child is kissing your baby or your nipples, or changing your baby's nappy and not washing their hands, they may be passing the infection back to you. It's worth them being checked by a doctor – and treated, if necessary.

Other causes of painful nipples

Mothers who suffer from skin conditions such as eczema and psoriasis can find that their nipples become sore while they are breastfeeding. If this is the case for you, you will need to discuss the problem with your GP or dermatologist so that you can find a treatment that is safe for your baby. A herpes infection of the skin on or near the nipple may mean that breastfeeding has to be suspended on that breast until the affected area has healed (see page 145 for information on how to stop breastfeeding temporarily).

Raynaud's phenomenon (also called Raynaud's syndrome), in which blood circulation to the extremities is poor, is a rare cause of painful nipples. People with this condition often find their fingers blanching, especially in cold weather – and some mothers discover that their nipples are also affected. The nipples will often look white after a feed and the most severe pain tends to occur when the blood rushes back into them as the baby lets go. Ineffective attachment makes the problem worse because pinching the nipples forces blood out of them. There is no cure for the phenomenon itself but your doctor can prescribe a specific drug for the pain. Keeping the breasts and nipples warm and ensuring effective attachment will also help.

Engorgement – why it happens and what to do

Engorgement is the painful swelling of the breasts that follows prolonged overfullness. The breasts feel hard, they may be inflamed (red) and the skin is often shiny. **If engorgement isn't dealt with quickly, milk production will start to slow down.**

Engorgement happens if feeding is not effective, feeds are cut short or there is a longer gap than usual between feeds. It is most common in the early days, when mother and baby are learning new skills and the breasts are working out how much milk is needed, and it's especially likely to happen if overfull breasts are ignored. ('Third day engorgement' was thought to be inevitable in the days when mothers and babies were separated in hospital and feeds were strictly timed but it's now known that these practices actually *caused* the problem.)

Effective attachment, frequent feeding and making sure your baby comes off the breast by himself are the keys to preventing engorgement (remember **FEEDS**, page 71). Being aware how your breasts feel between feeds, and offering your baby a feed – or expressing some milk – if they begin to feel heavy will help you to avoid engorgement.

The best way to relieve engorgement is to feed your baby. However, hard, swollen breasts make attachment difficult. You can help him by hand expressing some milk (see page 86) to soften your breast before he feeds. If you are still uncomfortable after he's fed (or if he isn't keen to feed) you will need to express some more milk (either by hand or with a pump) to relieve the fullness. There's no need to try to empty your breasts (breasts are never really empty, since milk is constantly being made); just express until you feel comfortable. If you want to, you can freeze the milk in case you need

YOU DON'T NEED CABBAGE LEAVES IN YOUR BRA!

An old 'cure' for engorgement was for mothers to put raw cabbage leaves over their breasts, inside their bra. It's not clear how this worked but it did seem to help. Nowadays we know it's much more important to remove some of the milk – which relieves the discomfort quickly *and* maintains milk production – than to walk around with a bra full of wilting vegetables.

it in the future (see page 150). If you have an older child who is still breastfeeding, they may be able to attach more easily than your baby – or you could ask your partner to 'feed'.

Although engorged breasts feel as though they are bursting with milk, it doesn't always flow readily. This is partly because the swelling in the breast narrows the ducts and partly because it reduces blood flow (so the oxytocin can't get through). Soaking in a warm bath or shower, or putting warm flannels on your breasts before feeding or expressing, can help to expand the blood vessels and enable the let-down reflex to work.

'My sister got really engorged and her baby couldn't latch on. She was holding her arms away from the sides of her body – her boobs were that sore. The breastfeeding support line said to put warm flannels on and do hand expression. She did one side and I did the other – there was loads of milk! Then all of a sudden she grabbed a breast in each hand and said "Thank God – they're mine again!" And half an hour earlier she'd barely been able to touch them at all.'

Jennifer, mother of Rebecca, eight years, and Nathan, five years

Blocked ducts – why they happen and what to do

A blocked (or plugged) milk duct feels like a small, hard lump in the breast. It's usually an irregular knotty shape, rather than smooth and round. It develops when something stops the milk moving smoothly through the duct. This can be as simple as a too-tight bra or a finger pressed into the breast during a feed. It can also happen if the baby is held in a way that prevents him from feeding effectively. Holding your baby in a different position for feeding once or twice a day can help to prevent ducts getting blocked.

At first, a blocked duct is painless so you won't notice it unless you feel for it. Then, as milk builds up behind the blockage, it will start to feel tender. If it isn't dealt with it can turn into mastitis (see page 240), so it's not something to ignore. **If you get into the habit of having a quick feel for lumps once a day, you'll be able to deal with problems as they arise.** Checking after a feed will give you the best picture because breasts sometimes feel slightly lumpy just beforehand.

Some women are more prone to blocked ducts than others, possibly because they have one or more ducts with kinks or narrow sections in them. Kinky ducts can be a quirk of nature or they can be the result of an injury or surgery to the breast. You can still breastfeed if you have a tendency to blocked ducts; you'll just need to check for lumps frequently.

Most blockages occur inside the breast but ducts can also become blocked where they open at the tip of the nipple. It's not clear what causes this but it seems that a micro-thin, transparent layer of skin forms over the opening. The milk that is dammed up shows through, appearing as a white spot or blister (sometimes known as a bleb) on the end of the nipple. This type of blockage often causes an intense, sharp pain (like a pin-prick), especially when the let-down reflex operates.

Wherever the blockage is, if it has been present for a while there may be a soft plug of thickened milk in the duct, similar to clotted cream. If your baby is feeding when the duct clears he will simply swallow the plug, but if you are expressing you'll probably see it emerge looking like a short piece of spaghetti.

How to clear a blocked duct inside the breast

Clearing a blocked duct within the breast is usually easy and painless. You can do it by hand, squeezing the area immediately *behind* the lump gently with your finger or thumb to express the plug, or you can help your baby to clear it while he's feeding:

- Find a position in which you are leaning forward over your baby, so that your breast is hanging free, away from your body. This allows gravity to help drain the milk. If possible, position your baby so that his chin (which does most of the work) is on the same side of the breast as the lump. You may need to be inventive to find a position that works – photos number 13 and 14 show two examples.
- As your baby feeds, gently massage the area over the blockage with your fingertips, using small, circular movements, until you can feel that the lump has gone.

How to clear a blocked duct at the end of the nipple

A duct that is blocked at the end of the nipple requires a slightly different approach because the seal needs to be broken to let the milk out. Here's how to do it:

- Sterilise a needle by boiling or by passing it through a flame; allow it to cool.
- Make sure your nipple is soft and warm. If necessary, drape a warm, wet flannel over it for a few minutes.
- Using the sterilised needle, gently pierce the white spot and lift the seal free. As long as you're careful, this won't hurt because there are no nerve endings in the seal.
- If the plug of thickened milk doesn't come out by itself, use your finger and thumb to squeeze behind the nipple and push it forwards.
- Continue expressing for a minute or two – or feed your baby, if he's willing – to be sure the blocked area is clear.

Mastitis – why it happens and what to do

Mastitis usually occurs in only one breast at a time. It's an inflammation, most commonly caused by an interruption to the normal flow of milk in one section of the breast, which then becomes hot and red – and very painful. It usually starts as a blocked duct (see above) but this stage can easily be missed because it doesn't hurt. If it isn't cleared, milk builds up behind the blockage and starts to seep out sideways, through the walls of the ducts – in the same way that damming a river will cause it to burst its banks. The surrounding breast tissue tries to deal with the problem by sending extra blood to the area. This is what causes the heat, redness and pain. If the milk in the affected area of the breast isn't helped to flow again quickly, the whole of the mother's body takes up the fight and she starts to feel as though she has flu – wobbly, sweaty and achy, with a raised temperature.

Mastitis can be accompanied by an infection, which usually needs to be treated with antibiotics. Unfortunately, the symptoms are the same whether there is an infection present or not, which means it's difficult to tell straight away whether antibiotics are needed. The important thing is to follow the treatment described below; if the mastitis is the non-infective type it will usually respond quite quickly. If it doesn't, it's likely there is an infection.

TIP

Mastitis can make breastmilk taste salty. Occasionally, the first sign that mastitis is brewing is the baby pulling off the breast and refusing to feed, because the milk tastes different. If your baby suddenly seems to dislike the taste of your milk, it's worth checking for lumps and redness.

Sometimes mothers with mastitis are advised to stop breast-feeding but this is *not* the best solution. **It's important to continue breastfeeding to clear the affected part of the breast – and your baby is the ideal person to help with that.** There's no risk of harming him through your milk and provided your doctor knows you want to continue to breastfeed, any medication they prescribe will be safe.

What to do if you have mastitis

Unless you have had mastitis before and know what to do, it's probably a good idea to consult your midwife or health visitor, or a breastfeeding specialist, so that they can support you while you treat the problem. You may also want to make an appointment to see your GP, so that you have a prescription for antibiotics on hand in case you need it (see below). But it's important not to waste any time before starting to deal with the problem yourself:

- Warm the sore breast with a hot shower or flannel – not scalding, but about the temperature you would normally use for bathing or washing.
- Encourage your baby to feed from that breast. Hold him so that he approaches your breast with his chin at the same side as the sore area, to give him the best chance of removing milk from that part. Make sure he's attached effectively (see page 50).
- If you can bear to touch the sore area, massage it with gentle strokes down towards the nipple while your baby is feeding, or put your hand flat against your breast and press slightly against that part, to help it to drain.
- Encourage your baby to feed frequently from the sore breast – at least every two hours, and preferably more often. If necessary, express the milk from your other

breast to keep it comfortable, so you can let him concentrate on the one with the problem.

- Try to rest and have plenty to drink. This won't have any direct effect on your breast but it will help to keep your fever down. Taking a simple anti-inflammatory medication, such as ibuprofen, will reduce the swelling and redness and help to reduce your temperature, too. (If you have a condition that means you can't take anti-inflammatories, paracetamol is a reasonable alternative.)

- If you don't start to feel better within six to eight hours you probably need antibiotics. If you haven't already got a prescription, see your doctor urgently. Make sure he or she knows you are breastfeeding (and want to continue), so they can choose the best medication for you.

- Continue with the warmth, frequent feeding and massage for a few days (with antibiotics, if you need them), until the soreness has completely gone.

'I was exhausted when I had mastitis. It was so painful, I couldn't do anything but lie on the sofa and feed. Arthur would feed for much longer than usual – it was as though he knew he had to clear it. Sometimes I'd lie down and get him to feed from over my shoulder so I could get his chin near the lump. Eventually you could see the lump going down as he fed. After that I'd get him to feed loads if I ever felt my breasts getting lumpy, just to head it off.'

Jemma, mother of Arthur, five years, and Rose, three years

If your baby isn't able or willing to feed frequently, your toddler (if he is still breastfeeding) may be able to help. If not, you'll need to express milk from the sore breast, either by hand or with a pump. Hand expression (see page 86) means you can target the sore part easily (with your thumb) but some women find using a pump (on a low setting), together with gentle stroking, is equally effective and more comfortable.

As well as treating the mastitis, it's important to try to work out what caused the problem, so you can correct it. Has your baby been feeding ineffectively? Has anything been digging into your breast or squashing it, either during or between feeds? Finding the cause will help to speed your recovery as well as preventing a recurrence.

Once the redness and pain have disappeared and you are feeling well again, you can go back to your baby's normal feeding pattern. Just make sure that he is attaching well, and check your breasts at least once a day.

If you think you have mastitis, don't just leave it and hope it will get better on its own. By not dealing with it you risk damaging your milk production – and, if there is an infection present and it isn't treated, there is a chance it could develop into a breast abscess.

Breast abscess – a rare complication

An abscess is like a large boil, which develops as the result of an infective mastitis that hasn't been fully dealt with. As with mastitis, the affected area of the breast will be hot and red, but it will also have what feels like a smooth, hard, round knob inside. This is because the pus that's produced can't drain and builds up in a sort of pocket. Breast abscesses are rare, but they are usually *extremely* painful.

What to do if you suspect a breast abscess

If you think you have an abscess, see your doctor urgently. He or she will almost certainly prescribe antibiotics and refer you for a specialist hospital appointment to have the abscess drained (this may need to be done more than once).

If the abscess isn't too close to your nipple, and you can bear to have your baby near that breast (did we mention it's usually *very* painful?), then you may feel able to keep feeding from it while it's being treated. If so, follow the treatment for mastitis, described on page 241. If you can't face it, continue feeding your baby from the other breast and do what you can to express the sore one, so that you don't become engorged. (This will also help to maintain milk production so that you can go back to feeding from both breasts when the abscess has cleared up.)

Once you've had a breast abscess you are likely to have some scar tissue inside your breast. This may make you more prone to blocked ducts (and mastitis) in that breast, so you'll need to be extra vigilant about your baby's attachment and about checking for lumps, both with this baby and with any future babies.

Stopping feeding from one breast, if you need to

If you are prone to problems such as mastitis, but find that it occurs only (or mostly) in one breast, you can decide to stop feeding completely from that breast while continuing to feed from the other one. Most women can produce plenty of milk for their baby from just one breast, so it's unlikely you will need to introduce any formula. If possible, choose a time when you are free from your recurring problem to make the change.

You can either wind down the feeding on the 'difficult' breast gradually or stop abruptly and express the milk instead. A gradual change will increase stimulation of the 'good' breast at the same time as giving the difficult one the message to reduce production. This will keep the total amount of milk available for your baby fairly constant. If you opt for the expressing method (see *How to stop breastfeeding quickly*, page 224), you will need to let your baby feed very frequently from the other breast for a couple of days to increase its production. In this case, you should try to avoid giving him too much of the milk you are expressing, so as not to dull his appetite. Unless you currently have a problem (such as mastitis) in the difficult breast, the gradual approach is probably the easiest.

The simplest way to begin a gradual changeover is to start offering the good breast first at each feed. As milk production in that breast increases you will be able to avoid offering the other breast at some feeds and milk production in that breast will begin to wind down. If you go a bit too fast and find the difficult breast gets uncomfortably full, just encourage your baby to feed from it once in a while, or express a little milk, until it settles down. After a couple of weeks you'll probably find you don't need to feed from the difficult breast at all.

Key points

- Breastfeeding shouldn't hurt. If it's painful you need to work out why and deal with it as soon as possible. Checking your baby's attachment is the best place to start.

- Creams and nipple shields won't prevent or cure damaged nipples – the answer is to make sure your baby is feeding effectively.

- Thrush is a fungal infection that can affect the nipples. It's easily passed between mother and baby; both need to be treated.

- Engorgement happens when feeding is not effective or frequent enough – or both.

- A blocked duct is easy to detect and to treat. Checking your breasts regularly for lumpy areas (preferably after a breastfeed) will help you to avoid painful breast conditions.

- Mastitis doesn't mean you have to stop breastfeeding – and it doesn't always need to be treated with antibiotics.

14

Breastfeeding
and illness

Continuing to breastfeed if either you or your baby is ill is important, both for health reasons and for emotional support. However, illness can make breastfeeding challenging – whether it's needing to use a different position if your baby has a cold or thinking about how to keep breastfeeding going if one of you has to be in hospital.

This chapter explains how to adapt breastfeeding around everyday illnesses, as well as providing some tips for coping with more serious conditions.

Breastmilk is the best food if your baby is ill

If your baby is ill, breastmilk is the best food and drink for her. It contains antibodies to help her fight infection – both the germs that are making her ill and others that might make her worse. It's also packed full of easy-to-digest nutrients. Older babies and toddlers often go off all their other food when they are poorly and want only breastmilk. (If you have stopped breastfeeding and want to start again because your baby is ill, see page 221.)

A change in your baby's feeding pattern may be the first sign you get that she is unwell. Typically, she will want lots of little drinks at the breast, rather than longer feeds. This may be because:

- She is thirsty.
- She has a raised temperature.
- She is lacking energy.
- Breastfeeding is difficult or painful (for example, if she has a blocked nose, a sore mouth or earache).
- She finds it comforting.

Experimenting with different positions may allow your baby to feed more comfortably. For example, an upright position will help mucus to drain and may make breathing easier if she has a cold, and prevent pressure on her ears if she has an earache.

If you continue to follow your baby's lead with feeding, your body will adjust your milk production to meet her needs. However, if she feeds less often than usual when she is ill you may find that your breasts get overfull. (This can also happen in the period immediately after the illness if she has fed very frequently during it.) Expressing some milk whenever you feel uncomfortable will help you to avoid engorgement and keep your milk production going at its usual rate. If your baby is under two weeks old and unable to feed frequently because of illness, you will need to express your milk as well as feeding her, so that the setting-up of your milk production is not interrupted.

Why skin-to-skin contact is good for an ill baby

Skin contact can be very comforting for an ill baby. It can also help to keep her temperature stable, by warming her up if she's cold and cooling her down if she's too hot. Don't be surprised, though, if holding your baby skin to skin when she's ill makes *you* feel hot – that's a sign that you're taking away some of her excess heat.

> ## TIP
>
> A moist atmosphere can make feeding easier for a baby with a blocked nose or sinuses, or a wheezy chest. Try feeding in the bathroom with the shower running hot, or in a warm bath together. A vapour rub applied to your breast near where your baby's nose rests when she's feeding (but not too close to your nipple) can also help.

'The way I produced more milk when Dayna needed it was amazing. If she was ill she'd go off her food completely and want nothing but cuddles and breastmilk. There always seemed to be loads for her almost as soon as she started feeding – even when she was a toddler. As long as she was sucking, my breasts would make milk, without fail.'

Barbara, mother of Dayna, five years

Ill babies sometimes need medicine or other treatment as well as breastmilk, so it's always a good idea to get your baby checked by a doctor if she is unwell – and to take her back to the doctor if she seems to be getting worse. This is especially important if she is vomiting, has a raised temperature or a rash, is wheezing, or seems listless or lethargic.

What if my baby is vomiting and has diarrhoea?

Sickness bugs and gastroenteritis are rare in babies who are fed solely on breastmilk. Breastfed babies are *meant* to produce lots of runny, yellow stools (see page 98) and, while her poo may occasionally have a slightly different smell or colour, as long as your baby is her usual self this isn't a cause for concern. However, if her pooing pattern is different from usual and she is vomiting (as opposed to possetting – see page 82), then she may have a stomach infection.

Vomiting and diarrhoea can quickly lead to dehydration, so it's important to get your baby seen by a doctor. However, breastmilk will probably be all she needs to allow her body to get rid of what is irritating it and replace the fluid that is being lost. Keeping an eye on how many wees she's doing will help you to monitor how well hydrated she is (although this may not be easy if she is passing lots of watery poo).

Babies don't need any extra water when they have a tummy upset. Breastmilk contains plenty of water, especially when feeds are short and frequent. Very short feeds are more likely to keep vomiting at bay than larger feeds, and feeding your baby in a position which makes it easier for her to control the flow of milk (see *If your milk flows too rapidly for your baby*, page 80) can help, too.

Animal milks (for example, cow's, goat's and sheep's milk) can irritate the stomach lining, so the usual advice is to avoid them – and products based on them, such as infant formula – if the stomach is already inflamed. This doesn't apply to breastmilk. Human milk is gentle on the stomach and it contains important growth factors to help the gut repair itself. In some cases, a special replacement drink (called oral rehydration therapy or ORT) may be prescribed in addition to breastmilk but there is no need for breastfeeding to stop. Even when a baby needs intravenous fluids, she can usually continue to drink breastmilk.

What if my baby needs an operation?

If your baby needs surgery her feeding will probably be disrupted – either just during the operation, or possibly for quite a bit longer.

If the surgery is planned it's a good idea to visit the ward where your baby will be cared for so you can talk to the staff in advance. For example, you'll probably want to find out whether you'll be able to sleep next to her and whether there are facilities for you to express and store your breastmilk on site. Paediatric ward staff don't always have much experience of breastfeeding, so you may need to explain what you need in some detail.

If your baby needs an anaesthetic, ask the staff how late her last breastfeed before the operation can be, so that you can make sure you offer her the chance to have a feed as close to it as possible. Breastmilk passes through the stomach very quickly (and is non-irritant), so it's usually allowed nearer to the operation than formula milk or any other food.

If the operation is a minor procedure, breastfeeding may be able to continue uninterrupted. If there has to be a slightly longer than usual gap between feeds, expressing some milk will stop you getting overfull. On the other hand, a long, complex procedure with complicated after-care may mean that breastfeeding isn't possible for several days. In that case expressing your milk will be very important, both to provide your baby with milk if she needs it while she is recovering and to maintain your milk production until she can start feeding again. See page 145 for information on expressing milk during a temporary break in breastfeeding.

Worrying about your baby can temporarily affect your let-down reflex, so if you are expressing milk, you may need to help the reflex to work (see page 147). If you have been able to express some milk in the days and weeks beforehand and freeze it at home, you'll have it to fall back on if necessary. Just knowing it's there will help to make the situation less stressful.

Breastfeeding is an effective pain reliever, especially where short-term painful procedures are concerned. **Research has shown that babies are soothed by being held, by skin-to-skin contact, by sweet tastes and by sucking. Breastfeeding combines all of these.** Just one word of caution, though: if your baby needs to have repeated painful procedures (such as blood tests), it may be best to breastfeed her immediately *after* the procedure rather than during it, just in case she starts to associate breastfeeding with pain and begins to refuse the breast (see page 103).

If your baby can't be picked up or is unable to move easily – perhaps because she has a drip or is in traction – you'll need to be inventive about how you feed her. As long as you can offer her your breast in a way that enables her to scoop it up effectively (see Chapter 3), it doesn't matter how you achieve this. Don't be afraid to ask for help from a member of staff and to move furniture and use cushions to help you get close to her at an angle that will work.

Parents of very ill babies sometimes feel powerless to help their child when she is in hospital, especially if she needs specialised care. Continuing to breastfeed your baby in this situation means you will be helping her in a way that no one else can – giving her the best nourishment she can have, and comforting her in a unique and special way.

'Saba needed heart surgery when she was eight months old. She wasn't able to feed for a few days afterwards so I had to express some milk. I'd never had a problem expressing before but I could hardly get anything. I think all the stress affected my let-down. When she came home, I relaxed a bit and we had lots of cuddles skin-to-skin and frequent feeds, and it was soon sorted.'

Shazia, mother of Jamal, six years, and Saba, four years

Can I keep breastfeeding if I'm ill?

Breastfeeding mothers are often advised – by family and friends, and sometimes by health professionals – to stop breastfeeding if they become ill. Sometimes this is because of unfounded fears about passing on the illness through the breastmilk and sometimes it is in the mistaken belief that producing milk drains a mother's energy and will make her illness worse. However, there are very few situations in which stopping breastfeeding is either necessary or a good idea.

Breastfeeding reduces stress, boosts a mother's immunity and stabilises her metabolism. **Breastfeeding women sleep better and get more nourishment from their food than women who are not breastfeeding, and they recover more quickly from common illnesses.** There are only a very few illnesses that can be passed on through breastfeeding and these are quite rare (HIV, for example, can sometimes be passed via breastmilk). So continuing to breastfeed is normally in the interests of both the baby and her mother.

What if I have an infection?

Most common infections, such as colds and tummy bugs, are passed from mother to baby through touching, kissing and breathing on one another, not through breastfeeding. And, while a formula feed can be contaminated as it's being prepared, this can't happen with breastmilk. If you have an infectious illness, your baby will already have been exposed to the germs that caused it before you know you are ill, so by continuing to breastfeed you will be helping to protect her from it – and to get better, should she catch it.

In the case of some infections – chickenpox, for example – it can be advisable for the baby to be given an immunisation but there is no reason for a mother who has chickenpox (or shingles, which is related to chickenpox) to stop breastfeeding.

Sometimes a mother who is ill simply feels too unwell to continue breastfeeding. However, it's important to bear in mind that stopping breastfeeding suddenly can lead to engorgement or mastitis (see Chapter 13) and, although expressing will help to prevent this, it may prove more awkward and difficult than continuing to breastfeed. It may be more helpful for someone to help you to breastfeed your baby than for them to give her a bottle.

Breastfeeding can help with postnatal depression

There is a widespread assumption that mothers who have postnatal depression shouldn't breastfeed. This seems to have arisen either because some people believe that breastfeeding makes PND worse or because they think depressed mothers need to be relieved of the 'burden' of feeding their babies. Neither of these beliefs is true. In fact, breastfeeding *reduces* the chances that a mother will develop PND – and if she does become ill, continuing to breastfeed will make some aspects of the illness easier to cope with.

Postnatal depression can make it hard to enjoy your baby or feel close to her; it can also make sleeping difficult. Breastfeeding can help with both these problems. The hormones released during breastfeeding will promote bonding and help you to relax, so although you may have to feed your baby more often – during the day and at night – you are likely to feel more rested and closer to her if you keep breastfeeding than if you switch to formula.

However, postnatal depression can make it difficult to tune in to your baby, which may mean that you don't always spot her feeding cues, especially if they are very subtle. You may also find it hard to pay attention to how effectively she is feeding when she's at the breast. If you have a supportive partner, close friend or family member, they may be able to help you make sure your baby is feeding effectively and frequently.

If you are finding mothering difficult, breastfeeding may be a key way of helping you feel that you matter to your baby, because it's something that only you can do. And if you have postnatal depression, helping you to continue breastfeeding is one of the most valuable things your partner, family and friends can do – for you *and* your baby.

'I started getting postnatal depression when Jacob was about five months old. Everything was overwhelming, and I felt inadequate as a mum. But I never lost my bond with Jacob – I didn't feel distanced like some mums who have it. I think breastfeeding was really important for that – it was comforting for me as well as him. In a world where everything was turned upside down, breastfeeding seemed to anchor us.'

Ruth, mother of Jacob, three years

The majority of drugs for postnatal depression are safe for breastfeeding mothers to take. However, your doctor may want to prescribe medications that he or she believes are particularly effective but which are not recommended during breastfeeding, and advise you to change to formula so that you can take them. It may help to have a supportive partner, friend or relative with you to help you explain why it is important for you to carry on breastfeeding, and to urge your doctor to choose an alternative drug.

What if I need to take medication?

Most medicines are safe to take while breastfeeding (see page 133). For the few that aren't, an alternative is usually available. However, some groups of drugs are almost always unsafe for breastfeeding babies. They include drugs for the treatment of cancer (chemotherapy). Radioactive compounds, injected for use in x-ray investigations, can also be harmful. In some cases it is not safe for the mother to feed or even hold her baby for several hours after the procedure, until the radioactivity has worn off.

If you are told you need to undergo an x-ray investigation involving the use of a radioactive compound, or take a drug which is not safe for your baby, try to find out whether it can be postponed, if only to allow you to stockpile some breast-milk in advance. If you will be able to resume breastfeeding after the procedure or course of medication, you'll need to express to keep yourself comfortable (and to keep your milk production going) while you can't breastfeed. See *What happens if I need to leave my baby for more than a day?*, page 145, for how to do this.

What happens with breastfeeding if I have to go into hospital?

Keeping your baby fully breastfed while you are in hospital isn't easy but it can be done – provided none of your drugs or treatments make your breastmilk harmful for your baby. Non-emergency admissions are obviously easier to manage than emergency ones, because they allow you to express and freeze some milk and discuss your needs with the hospital staff in advance.

Try to negotiate a single room, with relaxation of the visiting hours, so that your baby can spend as much time with you as possible without being exposed to too many germs. You may be able to borrow a breast pump from the maternity or neonatal unit, or hire one from an organisation such as the NCT (see page 278). Make sure the fact that you are breastfeeding is recorded in your hospital notes.

If you are going to have an operation, aim to feed your baby or express your milk as close as possible to the time you go to the operating theatre, to minimise the discomfort of very full breasts afterwards. Make sure that all the doctors involved in the operation (including the anaesthetist) know you are breastfeeding. Unless they tell you otherwise, it will be okay for you to breastfeed as soon as you are awake, provided someone is there to help you hold your baby.

Key points

- Breastmilk is the perfect food for your baby if she is ill. It contains antibodies to fight infection, it's easily digested and it won't irritate her tummy.

- A change in your baby's normal feeding pattern can be an early sign that she is ill. Poorly babies often want to have lots and lots of short feeds.

- Skin-to-skin contact can be helpful in regulating your baby's temperature.

- If your baby has an ear or chest infection, or a cold, you may have to change your usual feeding position to make it easier for her to feed.

- Frequent, small feeds will help to prevent dehydration if your baby has sickness and diarrhoea.

- If your baby needs an operation, try to plan ahead so that you can express and breastfeed while she is in hospital.

- If you are ill, continuing to breastfeed will benefit both you and your baby.

- If you have postnatal depression, breastfeeding can help you to sleep better and to enjoy your baby.

- Some investigations and drug therapies mean breastfeeding has to be interrupted but they rarely mean it has to end.

- If you need to be in hospital, talk to the staff about having your baby with you. If possible, express some milk in advance, so that you have it in reserve.

15

Conditions that make breastfeeding difficult

Sometimes physical or medical conditions can make breast-feeding extra challenging but it's very rare that it can't happen at all. Whatever the circumstances, you and your baby still have most, if not all, of the basic abilities and instincts for breastfeeding to be baby-led, even if you can't use all of them in quite the same way. While it's important for you both to have help with the things you can't do, it's just as important that neither of you is prevented from doing the things you can.

This chapter looks at how conditions such as cleft lip/palate, low muscle tone, cardiac (heart) and breathing problems can affect a baby's ability to breastfeed and suggests ways to help you and your baby work around the difficulties. (For more on the effects of illness, drugs and surgery on breastfeeding, see Chapter 14.)

Helping your baby to get milk easily

When feeding is ineffective, it's tiring for the baby and may not provide enough stimulation for the mother's breasts. If your baby has a weakened ability to suck, as well as helping him to feed as effectively as he can (see below), you may need to express after and/or between feeds to ensure that your breasts make plenty of milk. This will help him to get milk with the minimum of effort, as well as ensuring long-term production. *How to give your breasts a two-week 'wake-up call'* on page 189 will help you to maximise the stimulation you give your breasts when expressing.

Breastfeeding if your baby has a cleft lip/palate

A cleft lip and cleft palate can occur singly or together. Sometimes there is a cleft in the gum as well. Either condition can present a real challenge because it interferes with the way the baby attaches to the breast and how efficiently he can suck. However, even if full breastfeeding is not possible, there are several reasons why babies with a cleft benefit from some breastfeeding, and from being given breastmilk.

Babies with cleft palates have an opening in the roof of their mouth, so that the mouth and the nasal cavity are connected. This means they often get milk leaking into their nose while they feed; breastmilk is much less irritating to the lining of the nose than formula. They are also prone to ear infections, which breastmilk can protect against. Breastfeeding helps to strengthen the muscles of the upper lip and palate, which will promote healing after surgery and aid eating and speech development later.

Surgery to repair a cleft lip is usually carried out while the baby is quite young. Breastfeeding is normally possible as soon as the effects of the anaesthetic have worn off. There is no risk to the stitches from feeding, although the area will probably feel tender at first. Surgery to repair a cleft palate is not usually carried out until the baby is a few months old; keeping breastfeeding going until that point can be challenging so it's a good idea to muster all the support you can from friends and family.

If your baby has a cleft lip

Having a cleft lip interferes with the baby's ability to form a seal around the breast. If there is no seal there will be only limited suction, so breastfeeding will be inefficient and tiring. A small cleft may be able to be filled by the breast, provided it's not too full and can mould itself to the shape of the baby's lip. Feeding your baby frequently, and expressing some milk before the feed, if necessary, will help to keep your breasts soft and pliable. If the cleft is too big to be filled by the breast itself, you may be able to use your finger or thumb to seal the gap while he feeds. Experimenting with different feeding positions will help you to find what works best for you both.

If your baby has a cleft palate

The cleft may be in the soft palate, the hard palate, or both. A cleft palate causes problems for breastfeeding in three ways:

- The cleft prevents a seal being formed around the breast within the mouth, so suction is limited.
- Milk can leak into the baby's nose during feeding.
- If the cleft involves the hard palate, there may not be a firm surface for the baby's tongue to press the breast against.

In addition, babies with cleft palate are inclined to hold their tongue in the cleft and to be reluctant to stretch it forward to scoop up the breast. For all these reasons, full breastfeeding for a baby with anything other than a very small cleft is not likely to be possible. In that case you will be shown how to use a specially designed bottle and teat to give your baby supplementary feeds.

The following tips will help you to maximise your baby's effectiveness when feeding at the breast:

- Experiment with your breasts being either firm or soft during feeding, to find out which suits your baby best. Expressing some milk will soften your breast; using breast compression (see page 196) will make it firmer.
- Experiment with feeding positions. Holding your baby so that his head is higher than his chest will help to prevent milk leaking into his nose – for example, lying back with him on your tummy, or sitting upright with his legs straddling your thigh. (If you have a long back you may need to use pillows to raise him to the right level.)
- Experiment with support for your breast and/or your baby's jaw, to help him keep the breast deeply in his mouth. The 'Dancer' hand position (shown below) may help.

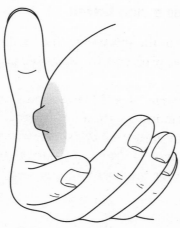

To support your baby using the Dancer hand position:

- Cup your hand under your breast, so that your last three fingers and part of your palm are supporting your breast and your thumb and forefinger are free.
- Open your thumb and forefinger to make a U shape. Bring your baby to your breast so that his chin rests in the centre of the U. Touch the pad of your forefinger

to one of his cheeks and the pad of your thumb to the other.

- Continue to support his jaw with gentle pressure on his cheeks throughout the feed. Take care not to prevent his jaw from moving up and down.

Breastfeeding if your baby has low muscle tone, heart or breathing problems

Babies with weak muscles, a cardiac (heart) condition and/or breathing problems tend to have difficulty feeding, either because their jaw and tongue movements aren't effective or because they tire quickly. Yet breastfeeding is particularly valuable for these babies because of the protection it gives against chest infections, and because it is less disruptive to their breathing and heart rhythms than bottle feeding.

Breastfeeding is particularly valuable – but often dismissed – for babies with Down's syndrome, because it protects against bowel problems, to which they are prone, and strengthens the facial muscles and tongue, providing long-term benefits for eating and speech.

Babies whose muscles are weak or who lack energy need to be able to feed without too much effort. Feeding in an upright or semi-upright position will help your baby to co-ordinate swallowing and breathing. It's important to provide gentle support for his head, while still allowing him to tilt it backwards. It helps some babies to maintain their attachment at the breast and to suckle more effectively if gentle pressure is applied with a fingertip just under and behind their chin, in a rhythmic, scooping movement, or if their lower jaw is supported using the 'Dancer' hand position (see above).

Feeding can't be entirely led by a baby who tires easily, since he's likely to need encouragement to feed. Stimulating his rooting reflex by stroking his face, especially his nose and lips, will encourage him to open his mouth. Patting his lips gently with your finger before putting him to the breast may also help. Holding him in skin contact while he is asleep will mean you can move him towards your breast as soon as he begins to stir, helping to conserve his energy for feeding.

A breastfeeding supplementer (see page 219) may help your baby to get more milk for the same amount of effort. If he is not able to feed effectively at the breast, you will need to express milk after a feed and give it to him as a supplement, using a dropper or small feeding cup. Babies with breathing or heart problems may also benefit from 'hindmilk feeding' (see page 192) to help them gain weight.

'Breastfeeding is like everything else with Down's syndrome babies – it takes longer for them to learn and you need to be extra patient and put in more effort. It was challenging in the beginning because Rana was so sleepy but it got better. It's worth it. She breastfed until she was two and she was always really healthy when she was little. I'm sure that was down to breastfeeding.'

Fahima, mother of Rafee, ten years, and Rana, eight years

Key points

- There are many health problems that can affect breastfeeding but they rarely mean it's impossible.

- It's worth seeking skilled, expert help from a breastfeeding specialist if you are facing a situation that will make breastfeeding unusually challenging.

Conclusion

Our aim in writing this book has been to provide you with practical information that will enable you and your baby to establish a happy and harmonious breastfeeding relationship and avoid the all-too-common problems that spoil the experience for so many families. We hope it has given you the knowledge and confidence to take a baby-led approach to breastfeeding, helping you and your baby to develop a strong and lasting bond.

The quick reference section that follows summarises some of the key information from the book. It includes the essentials of baby-led breastfeeding, what to expect as breastfeeding progresses and a quick symptom checker to help you track down the reason if you are finding breastfeeding painful.

We hope you have enjoyed this book and we wish you and your baby a rewarding and relaxed breastfeeding experience.

Quick reference

Baby-led breastfeeding – in a nutshell

Baby-led breastfeeding relies on you and your baby being in tune, so you can respond to her needs and she can help your breasts to make plenty of milk. If she's allowed to feed whenever she asks, you will be able to keep pace with her need for milk as she grows. However, it's important that she's able to attach effectively each time, so that she can get milk easily and give your breasts the right messages. This will also ensure breastfeeding is pain free for you.

In a nutshell, aim for breastfeeding to be:

- **F**requent – day and night.
- **E**ffective – with your baby attached so that she can get milk easily.
- **E**xclusive – your baby has only breastmilk – no other drinks or food (for the first six months).
- On **D**emand – whenever your baby asks, and for as long as she wants each time.
- **S**kin to skin as much as possible, in the early weeks.

Here's how to do it:

1) **Get to know your baby's feeding cues** so you can feed her before she gets upset. Offer her a feed *before* she asks, if your breasts are uncomfortably full.

2) **Get reasonably comfortable before the feed** but don't get too settled. Have a small cushion or a rolled-up jumper ready in case you need it. A snack and a drink is a good idea, too.

3) **Hold your baby in a way that will make feeding easy for her**, i.e. with:
   - as much of her body in contact with yours as possible
   - her whole body in line (with her knees and nose facing the same way)
   - her body weight supported (neck, shoulders and hips)
   - her head and arms free
   - her nose lined up with your nipple ('nose to nipple').

   Support your breast, if you need to.

4) **Give your baby time to attach** and start feeding. Help her by bringing her in *really* close, very quickly, when her mouth is at its widest (unless she's lying on top of you, in which case she'll do it herself). Make sure you don't have your hand on her head as you do this.

5) **When she starts to feed, check that:**
   - her chin is pressed into your breast
   - she has a wide-open mouth
   - her cheeks are full and rounded
   - more of your areola is showing above her top lip than below her bottom lip (if you can see any of it)
   - she is starting to suck in a rhythmic way, with a big yawning movement followed by a swallow.

6) **Decide what you need to do to be comfortable.** For example, use a cushion or rolled-up jumper to support your elbow or back. Relax and enjoy the feed.

7) **Let your baby feed for as long as she wants**. When she lets go of the first breast, offer her the second. Be ready to offer her the first again afterwards if she seems to want it. When she turns down the chance to re-attach, that's when she's had enough.

Breastfeeding this way will help you to make as much milk as your baby needs and ensure feeding is comfortable and relaxed.

Baby-led breastfeeding: what to expect when

It's a good idea to know what to expect as breastfeeding progresses, so you can either be reassured your baby is behaving normally or quickly spot any potential problems. If you think your baby is unwell, or you are struggling to care for him, contact your midwife, health visitor or GP. If you want specific help with breastfeeding you may prefer to contact a breastfeeding specialist (see *Where can I get help?*, page 106) or support organisation (see *Sources of information and support*, page 278). The grid below and overleaf outlines what you can expect, provided you and your baby are well.

When	What to expect – your baby	What to expect – you	What to do	Seek help if ...
First few hours	1 to 2 hours awake and alert, then a long sleep. Will find the breast on his own and have his first feed. NB: Wakefulness may be delayed if drugs are used in labour.	Exhausted but not sleepy (at first). Ready to get to know your baby.	Have uninterrupted skin-to-skin contact, at least until your baby has had his first feed.	

When	What to expect – your baby	What to expect – you	What to do	Seek help if ...
First 5 days	Number of feeds per day increasing, peaking on day 5. Gradually more wees. Poo changing from dark green/black meconium to runny yellow 'korma sauce' (see page 98). Small weight loss – no more than 10 per cent. Mild jaundice may develop from day 2.	Breasts gradually feel heavier as milk production gets going. May feel let-down reflex as tingling; possibly some leakage. Milk changing from thick yellowish colostrum to whiter, less concentrated milk. Some nipple tenderness possible at the beginning of feeds. After-pains during feeds. You may be emotional and weepy ('baby blues') from day 3.	Keep your baby near you, day and night. Encourage your baby to breastfeed frequently, especially if you feel full. A lying-back position can help you both learn. Watch and listen to him feeding; notice his sucking and swallowing pattern. Learn to express your milk by hand.	... breastfeeding hurts beyond the first few seconds of a feed. ... your baby doesn't swallow after every 1 or 2 sucks. ... your breasts are engorged. ... your baby isn't weeing more each day. ... your baby's poo isn't changing colour.
5–15 days	Jaundice gradually fades (usually by day 7 or 8). Feeding frequent – probably 12 times or more in 24 hours; may be erratic. Birth weight regained. Frequent yellow poos.	Breastfeeding is pain free. Breasts feel full before feeds and softer afterwards. 'Baby blues' becoming less.	Keep your baby near you day and night. Encourage your baby to breastfeed frequently. Give only breastmilk. Avoid teats and dummies. Experiment with different feeding positions. Learn to feed lying on your side. Get into the habit of checking your breasts for lumpy areas once a day.	... breastfeeding hurts. ... your breasts are hard or lumpy. ... your baby isn't feeding *at least* 6 times a day. ... your baby isn't doing at least 6 wees and 2 poos each day.

When	What to expect – your baby	What to expect – you	What to do	Seek help if ...
2–6 weeks	Baby's own breastfeeding pattern emerging. Feeding 6–12 times a day (or more) – cluster feeding likely. Gradually becoming more adept at feeding. Poos may be less frequent from 4 weeks.	Breasts feel full before feeds and softer afterwards. Need to concentrate less when feeding.	Keep your baby near you day and night. Offer a breastfeed whenever your baby asks (or earlier). Give only breastmilk. Avoid using a teat until confident your baby is feeding effectively. If you want to use a dummy, keep use to a minimum.	... breastfeeding hurts. ... your breasts have a hard, red or lumpy area. ... your baby isn't feeding at least 6 times a day. ... your baby isn't doing at least 6 wees and 2 poos each day. ... your baby is still jaundiced.
6 weeks –3 months	Feeds may become shorter (as feeding gets more effective). Occasional 'appetite spurts' likely. Beginning to smile and communicate in new ways. May be long gaps between poos.	Breasts start to feel soft most of the time (unless there is an unusually long gap between feeds).	Keep your baby near you day and night. Offer a breastfeed whenever your baby asks (or earlier). Give only breastmilk. If you want to use a dummy, keep use to a minimum.	... breastfeeding hurts. ... your breasts have a hard, red or lumpy area.
3–6 months	Gradually more interested in surroundings. May not want to focus on feeding. Occasional 'appetite spurts' likely. Possibility of teething.		Keep your baby near you day and night. Offer a breastfeed whenever your baby asks (or earlier). Give only breastmilk. If you want to use a dummy, keep use to a minimum.	... breastfeeding hurts. ... your breasts have a hard, red or lumpy area.

When	What to expect – your baby	What to expect – you	What to do	Seek help if ...
6–9 months	Interested in handling and tasting solid foods and trying new ones; may eat small quantities. Poo may contain small pieces of solid food. Teething likely; the odd nip a possibility.		Offer a breastfeed whenever your baby asks (or earlier). Let your baby know that you don't want to be bitten (learn to intercept when it's about to happen). Invite your baby to join in your mealtimes and begin to explore solid foods.	... breastfeeding hurts. ... your breasts have a hard, red or lumpy area.
9–12 months	May start to ask for fewer or shorter breastfeeds. Enjoys a range of foods. Eats something at most mealtimes. Feeds himself efficiently with his hands. May want to try using cutlery.	Milk production may begin to lessen, especially if baby has drinks of water.	Offer a breastfeed whenever your baby asks (or earlier). Include your baby in as many family mealtimes as possible.	... breastfeeding hurts. ... your breasts have a hard, red or lumpy area.
12–36 months and beyond	Breastfeeds becoming less frequent – but just as enjoyable and special. Using spoon and fork with food more efficiently.	Milk production gradually declines as child feeds less often.	Offer a breastfeed whenever your baby asks – or negotiate timings with your toddler. Continue breastfeeding for as long as both you and your child are enjoying it.	... breastfeeding hurts. ... your breasts have a hard, red or lumpy area.

Painful breastfeeding: quick symptom checker

Breastfeeding shouldn't hurt. If it *is* painful, the grid overleaf will help you to identify what's wrong and point you to where you can find more information in the book. **If you can't resolve the problem yourself, seek specialist help** (see *Where can I get help?*, page 106). Bear in mind it's quite common for more than one problem to occur at the same time, especially where the root cause is the same.

Where the problem is	Appearance	Feeling	Likely diagnosis
One or both nipples	Nipples may be slightly pink or red.	Pain at the beginning of a feed in the breast being used.	Initial attachment not ideal but baby quickly adjusts.
One or both nipples	Nipples misshapen when baby lets go and may appear white or blue-ish. Otherwise nipples red, may be cracked and bleeding.	Pain throughout a feed, which stops when the baby lets go. Nipples may be painful to touch.	Ineffective attachment lasting throughout feed.
One or both nipples and areolas May be deep breast pain.	Nipples and areolas may appear pink and/or shiny.	Sharp or burning pain throughout a feed, which continues (or worsens) when the baby lets go.	Thrush infection
Both breasts (commonly behind the nipple)	Nipples and breasts not inflamed, damaged or sore.	Short-lived pain soon after the beginning of a feed, accompanied by leakage of milk or sudden increase in baby's swallowing.	Painful let-down reflex
One or (usually) both breasts	Breast(s) shiny and swollen. May be red. Swelling may extend into armpit(s).	Breast(s) feels hard to the touch. May have raised body temperature.	Engorgement
Usually one breast	White spot visible at tip of nipple.	Pain, especially during feeds. May be tender to touch.	Blocked duct near nipple opening (white spot)
Usually one breast	Small, hard lump in breast.	May be pain, especially during feeds. May be tender to touch. But may be pain free.	Blocked duct within breast
Usually one breast	Hard, red area in breast, often wedge-shaped. May extend into armpit.	Severe pain, especially during feeds. May have raised temperature. May feel shivery and achy (flu-like).	Mastitis. If problem has existed a long time, may be an abscess.

Cause	Remedy
Baby not held close enough and/or encouraged to attach before mouth is open really wide.	Pull baby's bottom in closer. Wait for wide open mouth before encouraging attachment.
Baby being brought to breast at wrong angle and/or with neck or body twisted and/or not held close enough and/or encouraged to attach before mouth is open really wide.	Ensure baby held close, head and body in line, nose to nipple. Wait for wide open mouth before encouraging attachment (see page 37). A lying-back feeding position may help (see page 43). Ask a breastfeeding specialist to check attachment.
Infection with candida. May follow a course of antibiotics. May have been passed on by another family member.	Confirm diagnosis with breastfeeding specialist. Seek treatment for mother and baby (and possibly other family members). See page 234 for further remedies.
Rush of oxytocin causing squeezing of milk ducts. This is a normal part of breastfeeding (although not always painful).	Breathe slowly as pain peaks and subsides. Will become less noticeable after the first weeks (see page 24).
In early days: ineffective attachment and/or infrequent feeding or shortened feeds. Later: unusually long gap between feeds or stopping breastfeeding abruptly.	Feed when baby wants for as long as baby wants. Ensure effective attachment at all feeds (see page 49).
Unknown – may be ineffective attachment.	Express milk 'plug' from duct (see page 238). Ensure effective attachment at all feeds (see page 49).
Ineffective attachment. Pressure on the breast from tight bra, bikini top or other clothing.	Ensure effective attachment at all feeds (see page 49). Try a change of position. Leaning-over position may help (see page 239).
Ineffective attachment and/or long gap or shortened feed and/or pressure on breast from clothing or sleeping position. May involve infection, especially if nipple cracked or any pus visible.	Ensure effective attachment at all feeds (see page 49). Try a change of position. Feed baby more from sore breast. See page 241 for more remedies. May need antibiotics, and abscess will need to be drained.

Sources of information and support

Support with breastfeeding – UK

The UK has four **mother-to-mother support** organisations, each offering support and information about breastfeeding and a national telephone helpline. Some also offer local one-to-one support and group get-togethers. The BfN provides specialist information on drugs in breastmilk. These organisations are not equally active in all areas of the UK but it's likely one of them will have a group near you.

The Association of Breastfeeding Mothers (ABM)
abm.me.uk. National helpline 08444 122 949

The Breastfeeding Network (BfN)
www.breastfeedingnetwork.org.uk. National helpline 0300 100 0210

La Leche League GB (LLLGB)
www.laleche.org.uk. National helpline 0845 120 2918

The NCT (National Childbirth Trust)
www.nct.org.uk. National helpline 0300 330 0700

The NHS National Breastfeeding Helpline is staffed by volunteers from some of the above groups: 0300 100 0212

Some **local NHS health-care trusts** run breastfeeding clinics, staffed by trained workers and volunteers.

The Baby Café™ charity co-ordinates a network of breast-feeding drop-in centres run by healthcare practitioners and voluntary breastfeeding counsellors.
www.thebabycafe.org

Other UK sources of support or information on breastfeeding

The Health Promotion Agency for Northern Ireland has a website devoted to breastfeeding.
www.breastfedbabies.org

Lactation Consultants of Great Britain (LCGB) is the professional association for qualified lactation consultants. (You can expect to have to pay for the services of a lactation consultant.)
www.lcgb.org

NHS Choices website offers breastfeeding information and support.
www.nhs.uk/Planners/breastfeeding/Pages/help-and-support.aspx

The UNICEF UK Baby Friendly Initiative works with the health-care system to ensure high standards of care for pregnant women, mothers and babies. It offers an assessment and accreditation programme for maternity and neonatal units, community health services and university courses. You can find out from the UNICEF website whether or not your local hospital or community trust has a Baby Friendly award. This

site is also an excellent source of up-to-date information and research on breastfeeding.
http://live.unicef.org.uk/babyfriendly

The United Kingdom Association for Milk Banking is a registered charity that supports human milk banking in the UK. It shares expertise and good practice with milk banks and breastmilk donors.
www.ukamb.org

The Welsh Government has a section of its website devoted to breastfeeding.
http://wales.gov.uk/topics/health/improvement/pregnancy/breastfeeding

Support with breastfeeding – other English-speaking countries

La Leche League has branches in most countries of the world.
www.lalecheleague.org

The Australian Breastfeeding Association aims to educate and influence society about breastfeeding, and to support mothers to do it.
www.breastfeeding.asn.au

The New Zealand Ministry of Health has a section of its website devoted to breastfeeding.
www.health.govt.nz/yourhealth-topics/maternity/breastfeeding

Support for combining breastfeeding and work

Childcare.co.uk is a good place to start if you need any form of child care.
www.childcare.co.uk

The Department of Business Innovation and Skills produces a leaflet 'Pregnancy and work – what you need to know as an employee'.
www.bis.gov.uk

The Health and Safety Executive produces a leaflet 'A guide for new and expectant mothers who work'.
www.hse.gov.uk/mothers

Working Families aims to help working parents achieve a good balance between their responsibilities at home and at work.
www.workingfamilies.org.uk

Support for breastfeeding in public

The Breastfeeding Welcome Scheme aims to support mothers' right to breastfeed their babies when they are out and about. The website gives details of businesses and venues in various areas across the UK that have signed up to welcome breastfeeding.
www.breastfeedingwelcomescheme.org.uk

Further information on baby-led weaning

Baby-led Weaning: Helping your baby to love good food, by Gill Rapley and Tracey Murkett, published by Vermilion, 2008

The Baby-led Weaning Cookbook: Over 130 delicious recipes for the whole family to enjoy, by Gill Rapley and Tracey Murkett, published by Vermilion, 2010

The following websites may also be useful, along with the growing number of parenting forums and blogs that discuss this approach to introducing solid foods:
www.baby-led.com
www.rapleyweaning.com

General parenting support and information

Best Beginnings campaigns to give every baby the healthiest possible start in life.
www.bestbeginnings.org.uk

Bliss provides support and care to premature and sick babies and their families.
www.bliss.org.uk

The Cleft Lip and Palate Association (CLAPA) provides information and support for people with cleft lip and/or palate and their families.
www.clapa.com

The Down's Syndrome Association provides information and support for people with Down's syndrome and their families.
www.downs-syndrome.org.uk

The Fatherhood Institute works to produce a society in which all children have a strong and positive relationship with their father and any father-figures.
www.fatherhoodinstitute.org

The General Osteopathic Council has a list of registered osteopaths, including those who specialise in cranial osteopathy and are used to treating babies.
www.osteopathy.org.uk

Gingerbread provides advice and practical support for single parents.
www.gingerbread.org.uk

Maternity Action aims to promote the health and well-being of all pregnant women, their partners and children.
www.maternityaction.org.uk. Telephone helpline: 0845 600 8533.

The Multiple Births Foundation aims to improve care and support for multiple birth families.
www.multiplebirths.org.uk

Netmums is run by mums in conjunction with health professionals.
www.netmums.com

The NCT (see page 278) provides general information on birth and parenting, as well as on breastfeeding.
www.nct.org.uk

The Twins and Multiple Births Association (TAMBA) aims to help parents meet the unique challenges of multiple birth.
www.tamba.org.uk

About the authors

Gill Rapley has worked as a midwife and a health visitor. She has also been a voluntary breastfeeding counsellor and lactation consultant. More recently, she spent 14 years working for the UNICEF UK Baby Friendly Initiative, helping maternity and community health workers to implement good standards of care for mothers and babies. She and her husband have three grown-up children and live in Kent.

Tracey Murkett is a writer and journalist, and she is also a voluntary mother-to-mother breastfeeding helper. She lives in London with her partner and their daughter, now aged six.

Gill and Tracey are the authors of *Baby-led Weaning: Helping your baby to love good food* and *The Baby-led Weaning Cookbook*.

Acknowledgements

We would like to thank everyone whose ideas, experiences, comments and wisdom have helped to create this book. They include colleagues, clients, acquaintances and friends past and present – including those whose insights we didn't recognise for what they were at the time.

We are particularly grateful to Sue Ashmore, Claire Davis, Jessica Figueras, Emily Hussain, Hazel Jones, Wendy Jones, Derrick Murkett, Jules Robertson, Jacqui Stronach, Anne Strong and Anne Woods for valuable feedback on the manuscript and for insight, support and inspiration.

Thanks to Gaby Jeffs of Magneto Films for supplying wonderful photographs, and to all the families pictured. We are grateful to them for allowing us to share their special moments.

Thanks, also, to our long-suffering editors, Louise Francis and Gill Paul, for their patience and tolerance, and to our agent, Clare Hulton, who has believed in us from the beginning.

Finally, we would like to thank our families for their constant support while we were writing – for keeping us fed and watered, and putting up with our tantrums when things went wrong.

Photo Credits

Thanks to the families for permission to use the following photos (© Gaby Jeffs of Magneto Films):

Billie, Mike, Ottilie and Anna, newborn and eight weeks (photos 3, 4 and 30)
Roma and Artemis, eight weeks (photos 5, 6, 14, 20–24 and 34)
Munira, six weeks (photo 7)
Michaela and Jacob, five weeks (photo 11)
Bronwen and Layla, 12 weeks (photos 13, 26–28 and 31)
Nadine and Beatrice, six weeks (photos 15–19, 25 and 32)
Rachael, Valentine and Aaron, two and four weeks (photos 33 and 36)
Kamila and Natasha, 10 weeks (photo 36)
Tracey and Nathan, eight weeks (photo 38)

And thanks to the families who provided us with photos of:

Clare and Scarlett, newborn, © Nick Caro (photos 1 and 2)
Trudy, Derek and Noah, newborn (photo 12)
Julia, Cassia, three years, and Fabian, one year, © M Tomkins (photo 29)
Maja and Bella, 20 months, © Cliff Castle (photo 35)
Callista and Ivy, six months (photo 37)
Natalie and Jonah, 13 months, © Adam Inglis (photo 39)

Photos 8–10 reprinted with kind permission from NCT's *What's in a nappy?* leaflet, 2012. www.nct.org.uk

Tuesday, Nov 26, 2013 - 16:35
Borrower number: *********3721

---

ou have renewed 1 item

itle	Due	Fee
abies the umsnet guide	17/12 13	

---

ou unsuccessfully tried to renew 1 ems

itle	Due
aby-led reastfeeding how to ake breastfeeding	

his item was issued to you earlier day.

---

ou have no other items on loan

mount owing: NONE

---

ease note: This does not include
ny charges for overdue items which
ave not yet been returned

Thank you for using this service

Index

Also available from Vermilion by Gill Rapley and Tracey Murkett

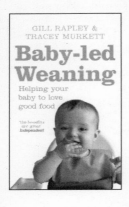

Baby-led Weaning

Exploding the myth that babies need to be spoon-fed, *Baby-led Weaning* shows how self-feeding from the start of the weaning process is the healthiest way for your child to develop. This book provides practical tips for getting started with baby-led weaning and the low-down on what to expect. No more purées and weaning spoons, and no more mealtime battles. Simply let your baby feed himself healthy family food.

£10.99   ISBN 9780091923808

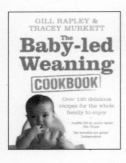

The Baby-led Weaning Cookbook

The Baby-led Weaning Cookbook offers comprehensive recipes and meal ideas that allow the entire family to eat together, to help your child become a happy and confident eater. Full of healthy, delicious meals and beautifully illustrated throughout, this book also includes simple advice on how to start, essential nutrition and safety information, ideas for quick snacks and lunches, as well as desserts and family dinners.

£12.99   ISBN 9780091935283

Order these titles direct from www.randomhouse.co.uk